ART PSYCHOTHERAPY GROUPS IN THE HOSTILE ENVIRONMENT OF NEOLIBERALISM

This book explores how 'the hostile environment' of neoliberalism affects art therapy in Britain. It shows how ambiguity in art and in psychoanalytically understood relationships can enable art psychotherapy groups to engage with class dynamics and aspire to democracy.

The book argues that art therapy needs to become a political practice if it is to resist collusion with a system that marginalises collectivity and holds individuals responsible for both their suffering and their recovery. It provides accounts of the contradictions that are thrown up by neoliberalism in art therapists' workplaces as well as accounts of art therapy groups with those affected by the fire at Grenfell Tower, in an acute ward, a women's prison, a community art studio and in a refugee camp.

Written by art psychotherapists for art therapists and other mental health workers, the book will bring political awareness and consideration of resistance into all art therapy relationships, whatever the context and client group.

SALLY SKAIFE, PHD, is an art therapist and group analyst working in mental health. She was a Senior Lecturer at Goldsmiths, University of London; a chair of the British Association of Art Therapists; a member of the editorial board of Inscape and, currently, ATOL; and has numerous publications.

JON MARTYN is an art psychotherapist and clinical supervisor. He was a lecturer at Goldsmiths College and co-founded the New Art Studio, a therapeutic art studio for refugees and asylum seekers with Tania Kaczynski. He now lives in Sheffield, South Yorkshire.

'This book is at the vanguard of the political turn taking place in sections of the psychotherapy profession. Eloquent and accessible, it is a powerful, critical account of how art psychotherapy has been used on "the front line" in a range of settings, not only to ameliorate the psychological harm produced by neoliberal policies, but also to empower the citizen. Skaife and Martyn's work is a call to arms, challenging many of the taken-for-granted norms of the psychotherapy profession.'

Farhad Dalal, *Psychotherapist and group analyst;*
Author of CBT: The Cognitive Behavioural
Tsunami: Managerialism, Politics and the
Corruptions of Science

'Sally Skaife and Jon Martyn's book comes at a critical moment as art therapists grapple with the impact of the neoliberal "free market" policies that have contributed to the vast divide between the rich and the poor. This book questions the impact of capitalism and marketization on the epistemology of art psychotherapy. Practicing art psychotherapy necessitates that we question our complicity in colluding with privatization that values profit over wellness. As the world comes to grips with the inadequate distribution of health care during COVID-19, which has severely impacted communities of color, this book should be necessary reading for anyone working in mental health.'

Savneet Talwar, *Professor; Chair, Department of Art*
Therapy, The School of the Art Institute of Chicago

'Just the title alone is sufficient for me to add this book to my "must read" list for 2021. The book summary promises a critical examination of art therapy in the context of a corporate capitalism that commodifies therapy and individualises distress and dis-ease, overlooking how social and institutional norms that are fundamentally unhealthy generate distress in the first place. Combining rigour with a fast and energetic polemical prose style, this book promises to be one of the most important (and I hope influential) art therapy texts of the decade.'

Susan Hogan, *Professor of Arts & Health*
University of Derby, College of Arts, Humanities
& Education; Professorial Fellow, Institute of
Mental Health, Nottingham

ART PSYCHOTHERAPY GROUPS IN THE HOSTILE ENVIRONMENT OF NEOLIBERALISM

COLLUSION OR RESISTANCE?

Edited by
Sally Skaife & Jon Martyn

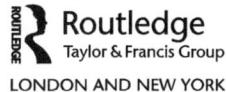
Routledge
Taylor & Francis Group

LONDON AND NEW YORK

Cover Image: 'Wounded Bear' by Andrew Mead

First edition published 2022
by Routledge
4 Park Square, Milton Park, Abingdon, Oxon, OX14 4RN

and by Routledge
605 Third Avenue, New York, NY 10158

Routledge is an imprint of the Taylor & Francis Group, an informa business

British Library Cataloguing-in-Publication Data
A catalogue record for this book is available from the British Library

Library of Congress Cataloging-in-Publication Data
Names: Skaife, Sally, 1952– editor. | Martyn, Jon, editor.
Title: Art psychotherapy groups in the hostile environment of neoliberalism : collusion or resistance? / edited by Sally Skaife & Jon Martyn.
Description: First edition. | Milton Park, Abingdon, Oxon ; New York, NY : Routledge, 2022. | Includes bibliographical references and index. |
Identifiers: LCCN 2021037739 (print) | LCCN 2021037740 (ebook) | ISBN 9780367619855 (hardback) | ISBN 9780367619848 (paperback) | ISBN 9781003107408 (ebook)
Subjects: LCSH: Art therapy. | Group psychotherapy. | Neoliberalism.
Classification: LCC RC489.A7 A7653 2022 (print) | LCC RC489.A7 (ebook) | DDC 616.89/1656—dc23
LC record available at https://lccn.loc.gov/2021037739
LC ebook record available at https://lccn.loc.gov/2021037740

ISBN: 9780367619855 (hbk)
ISBN: 9780367619848 (pbk)
ISBN: 9781003107408 (ebk)

DOI: 10.4324/9781003107408

Typeset in Minion Pro
by codeMantra

Dedication

'… for the many, and not the few …'

CONTENTS

CONTENTS

CONTRIBUTORS

Holly Caldecourt is a state-registered art psychotherapist. Holly holds a BA (Hons) in fine art from Central Saint Martins and an MA in art psychotherapy from Goldsmiths, University of London. She currently works for Latimer Community Art Therapy (LCAT), a grassroots organisation, and lives in London.

Annamaria Cavaliero is a British art psychotherapist working in adult mental health. Author of 'Considering the function of repetition in art and art psychotherapy', *ATOL: Art Therapy OnLine*, 7(1), 2016; and 'The breath and the line: An art therapist's subjective account of drawing through illness', *ATOL*: 12(1), 2021.

Jessica Collier is an art psychotherapist working for the NHS with women in prison in the UK. She has taught, lectured and published widely on forensic art psychotherapy, and is co-convenor of the Forensic Arts Therapies Advisory Group and co-editor of the *International Journal of Forensic Psychotherapy*.

Emily Hollingsbee is an artist and art psychotherapist. She works at a primary school and at New Citizens' Gateway, and is a team member at Art Refuge. Emily co-founded the not-for-profit organisation, Draw On, which offers workshops and art therapy groups to refugees, asylum seekers and migrants in the UK.

Beulah Lambert is an HCPC-registered art psychotherapist and clinical supervisor based in London. She works as a full-time art psychotherapist with children and young people in various settings, which have included pupil referral units, primary and secondary schools, and community centres.

Jon Martyn is an art psychotherapist and clinical supervisor. He was a lecturer at Goldsmiths, University of London and co-founded the New Art Studio, a therapeutic art studio for refugees and asylum seekers with Tania Kaczynski. He now primarily works in a private practice in Sheffield, South Yorkshire.

Katie Miller is an art psychotherapist and visual artist. She is an art therapist with Art Refuge and New Citizens' Gateway, working with unaccompanied children and young people. In 2019 she co-founded Draw On, which provides group art therapy to refugees, asylum seekers and migrants in the UK.

Helen Omand is an art therapist who works in a therapeutic art studio and teaches on the MA Art Psychotherapy programme at Goldsmiths, University of London. She is interested in the relationship between personal art practice and working as an art therapist, and exhibits with a collective of artists and art therapists.

Susan Rudnik is a registered UK Art Psychotherapist, clinical supervisor and lecturer. Qualifying in 2006, Susan has worked on paediatric wards in the NHS, in schools and in private practice. She teaches on the MA Art Psychotherapy programme at Goldsmiths, is on the editorial board of ATOL, and is founder and co-director of Latimer Community Art Therapy.

Sally Skaife (PhD) is an art therapist and group analyst working in mental health. She was a Senior Lecturer at Goldsmiths, University of London; a chair of the British Association of Art Therapists; and a member of the editorial board of Inscape and, currently, ATOL; and has numerous publications.

ACKNOWLEDGEMENTS

We would like to thank Dr Maia Kirby, Dr Robin Tipple and Dr James West, and our partners, Kat and Dave, for their wisdom, support and encouragement.

PART ONE

Resisting capture

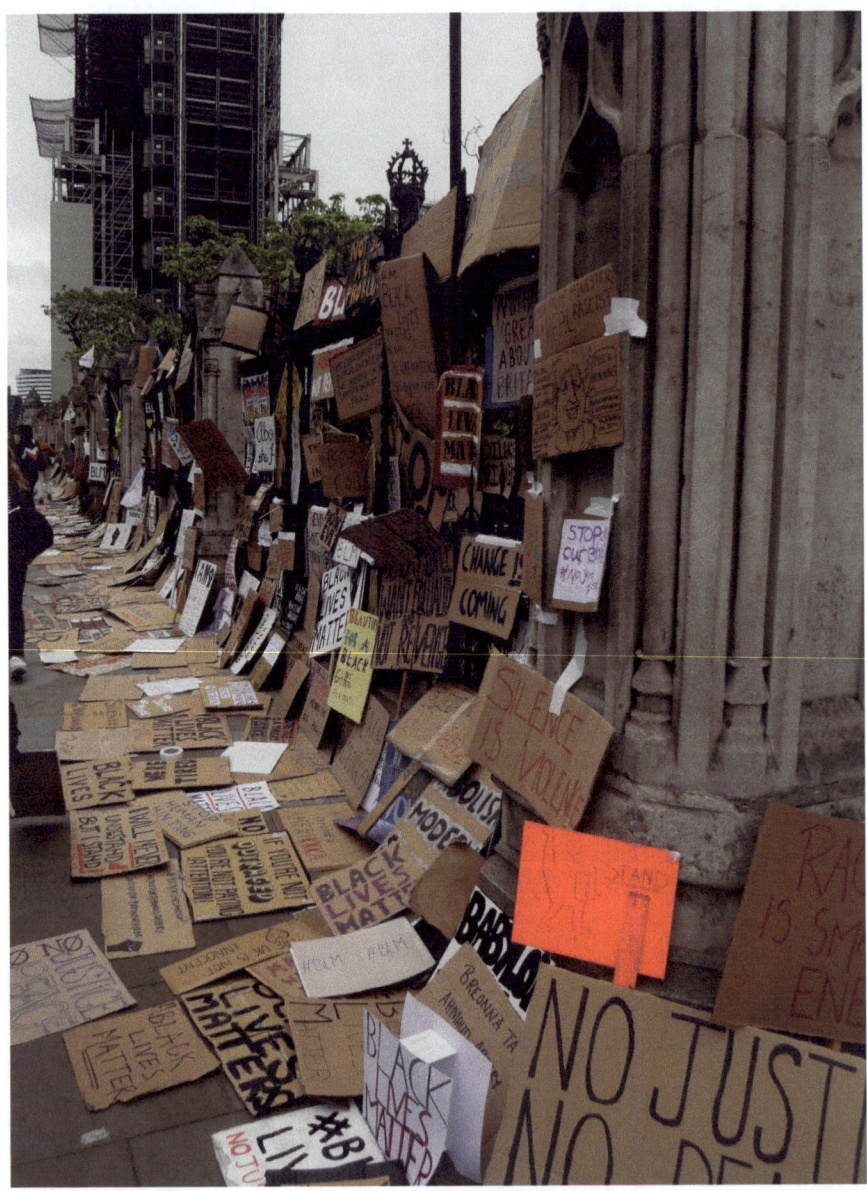

Figure P.1 *Placards left at the gates of the Houses of Parliament, London, after a Black Lives Matter demonstration in 2020. Photograph by Jon Martyn.*

CHAPTER ONE

The hostile environment

Sally Skaife and Jon Martyn

DOI: 10.4324/9781003107408-2

Neoliberalism has been with us for a while but now its own contradiction, that it profits only the few whilst it disadvantages the many, threatens humanity itself through climate extinction, wars and pandemics. Meanwhile, neoliberalist hegemony is having a disastrous effect on the mental health of the majority. This urgent situation requires art therapists to no longer ignore its contradiction, but how should we respond?

Over the last few decades it has become increasingly apparent that art therapy,[1] in adapting to the demands of the market within mental health services, has been persuaded to abandon some of the subversive and radical ideas that drove its development in the 1970s and 1980s. Art is constrained by treatment models as we are forced to ensure 'efficiency' by providing evidence, turning patients and art therapy packages into products for measurement. Our workplaces, where they still exist, often seem toxic and punitive – not only are 'patients'[2] made to fit a profit-making system based on the supposed neutrality of numbers, so too are we rated against performance targets. Other art therapists work alone, needing to sell their product to individuals experiencing alienation and in relationships tainted by an uncaring, racist, sexist, discriminatory society. The most difficult problem is that, as art therapists, we feel required to be in a state of disavowal, unable or unwilling to see things as they are, and so are liable to collude with the idea that the 'patient's' distress is because of a lack within them rather than in the social world, which we can treat or respond to through the market-led drive of wellbeing projects.

We live in an unjust world in which accelerating inequalities, associated with neoliberalism, have led to a few billionaires and transnational corporations, supported by governments, owning nearly all the wealth. They control the means of production and distribution, as well as the media and the military. Meanwhile, the majority in the world live in

---

1 Art therapy/art psychotherapy. We tend to use these terms interchangeably throughout the piece. This is a split we'd prefer to hold in a dynamic tension, rather than resolve.
2 Patient/client/service user are used interchangeably as we find none of these terms satisfactory, each having difficult connotations.

poverty and are subject to violence. Black[3] and people of colour are the worst off, and women are exploited for free care work and low-wage work, the Western world suffering less because it still profits from what was the colonised world. The capitalist system that creates this is lodged into all our institutions and services, and thus in our ideologies too, to the extent that it is difficult to imagine it could be any other way.

In this book, though, instead of being sunk by the neoliberalist contradiction, we recognise the potential in art therapy for subverting it. To survive contradictions, we repress what doesn't fit; the practice of art therapy provides the possibility for the representation of what becomes repressed and for engaging with mind/body splits that have been exploited by capitalism in racism, patriarchy and elitism (Skaife, 2013). Art holds ambivalence and contradiction, as do psychodynamically understood relationships, and we maintain that these can be tools through which we challenge the contradictions to which neoliberalism gives rise. In the book we consider how neoliberalism, with its methods of fragmentation, marketisation, commodification and disempowerment, has affected those with whom art therapists work, art therapists themselves, our profession, its training and art therapists' practice.

This introductory chapter and the two that follow in Part One, are contextual introductions to the seven contributor chapters in Parts Two and Three. In this chapter we introduce the book and discuss the effects of neoliberalism on society, focusing on the UK government's austerity regime and the effects of marginalisation. In Chapter Two we look at the way neoliberalism has invaded our institutions and led to a shift in our values. Chapter Three considers the way that art therapists have approached politics in their art therapy group practice. The seven contributor chapters show art therapists grappling with the difficulties of staying with the conflict and stress in the day-to-day work, recognising their own social position

---

3 Identifiers. We are unable to find satisfying terms for signifiers of identity. We recognise that the use of racial terms contributes to the positions of difference. Where the capitalised 'B' is used in regard to 'Black', this refers to political blackness; and is in recognition of class/colonial oppression of the many. Where other authors have used different terms, we have tended to use their terminology. When class is discussed, we have hoped for this to be an identifier which transcends racial constructs, such as 'the white working class'.

within it. Lastly, the Epilogue draws from all the chapters to consider art therapy groups as potential spaces of political action.

HOW THE BOOK BEGAN

The seed of this book began in 2018 when Jon was approached by a publisher to write an art therapy book in response to the European refugee crisis. The focus was to be, 'What resources are needed for art therapists working with refugees and migrants?' The question seemed to allude to, yet evade, a more important question: why is this 'population' denied access to resources and even the most basic rights? Jon felt somewhat uncomfortable writing a book that solely focused on refugees and the crisis. He was disquieted by the way migrants were described; they were often seen as a problem even from sympathetic sources and framed as victims which Europe's governments had a duty to save as individuals. The idea of writing about migrants seemed to feed into a process of marginalisation. Such frames focus the problem on the migrant and distract from the wider political agendas, that is, the creation of militarised territorial borders that, whilst allowing the unimpeded transit of capital, of goods and of the wealthy, violently exclude the movements of the poor, however desperate their plight. Jon approached Sally with this conundrum. We had both worked with the organisation that is currently called Freedom from Torture and on the MA Art Therapy training at Goldsmiths, and we shared an involvement with political activism.

In our early discussions we considered the idiom 'Hostile Environment' as a term that encompasses the way in which we are all affected negatively by neoliberalism. The term was coined in 2012 by the then home secretary, Theresa May, and referred to a set of administrative and legislative measures designed to make staying in the UK as difficult as possible for people without settled status in the hope that they might 'self deport'. We considered this a feature of a divisive culture that sets us against each other and projects suffering into one group of people, who can be nominally supported by another group, but the oppressive, disempowering system remains intact.

CONTRIBUTING AUTHORS

We had decided to invite art therapists to contribute chapters to the book who had a psychodynamic approach to their work with marginalised communities. Unsurprisingly, amongst this group were relatively new practitioners, opening a possibility for a fresh approach to art therapy work. We asked them to write about the effects of the hostile environment on their practice, about power differences that arise within the therapy, and to describe case material with attention to detail and to the specific. We were wanting authors to consider how political dynamics become replicated in their art therapy work, and how, as art therapists, they face the challenges presented by them. We thought that art therapists were finding themselves in an Alice in Wonderland world in which little made sense, and that if they were not to be totally sucked in, were in a state of continuous anxiety and stress.

We decided to embrace the subjective and consider the book as a whole as a reflexive practice, much like therapy and like making art, rather than attempt to provide an overall idea of the nature of provision of art therapy in a particular area. So, in asking our authors to address certain topics, we decided the field, they responded to this, and we responded to their drafts according to what we were learning as we were developing our thinking and learning from the authors. We hope that the book gives rise to thoughts that are also applicable to other areas of therapy work.

PSYCHODYNAMICALLY BASED ART THERAPY GROUP WORK

When we received the chapter proposals we realised that all the authors had written about group work, which then gave a particular focus to the book. Our own art therapy practices were predominantly in psychodynamically based art therapy group work and the training we had both taken and taught was based in the same. Sally had training in group analysis and had been conducting, writing and researching art therapy groups for many years. Jon has an ongoing interest in therapeutic communities, having worked within two before co-founding the New Art Studio, a therapeutic art studio for asylum seekers and refugees.

There are frequent criticisms of psychodynamically based art therapy in the art therapy literature that pick up on unquestioned power relations in psychoanalytic theory (Wood, 2011, Springham et al., 2012, Hogan, 2015, Talwar, 2018). We recognise the origin of psychoanalysis in middle class circles in Central Europe and the adoption of colonialist positions in relation to 'the other', which ascribe to the patient projections of 'the primitive', sexuality, aggression and so on. Also, the analyst's regard of themselves as experts on the patient's unconscious must be rejected. However, psychoanalysis came from Freud's radical philosophy in which human development was understood dynamically and as embodying contradictory notions, such as between nature and nurture (Blackwell, 2003). Understanding the mind/body binary dynamically allows us to appreciate how it has been exploited in social class, racism, patriarchy and in mental health provision, and in the way we work in art therapy (Skaife, 2001, 2013). We argue, like Blackwell (2003), that all therapy models are derived from psychoanalysis and similarly exhibit a power dynamic derived from colonialism. Those that attempt to police discriminatory attitudes within the therapy can be said to exert more power over 'the patient' than those that allow the unequal power dynamics, inherent in all our relations, to emerge and be thought about.

We were also aware that, though there is a radical tradition in art therapy in the therapeutic community movement and in the open studios in asylums which ran counter to traditional psychiatry, the political potential of groups is not always what is harnessed from them and they do not inherently solve the problem of the individualising of mental health and its market. Art therapy groups, too, have become packaged up as sets of techniques and sold to the representatives of diagnosed client groups. However, we consider that art therapy groups provide a field of social relationships that art can give form to, and art making can rework. Art offers a subversive, alternative communication which can upset our habitual language. We were influenced by the writings of de Maré et al. (1991) on the potential, in large groups, for moving away from hierarchical to democratic relating, considering the ideas also relevant to smaller groups. In groups that do not have an explicit agenda but let the process go as it will, the dynamics of the dominant culture, which are present within the hosting institution, will inevitably emerge. The reiterations of these dynamics in art making, performing, looking and talking can allow for new meaning; art therapy, then, can be politics in action (Skaife et al., 2020).

PLACING THE BOOK

After we had begun working on the book we discovered Savneet Talwar's ground-breaking book from Chicago, USA, which was asking similar questions to us (Talwar, 2018). She writes about the need for radical caring and social justice, and a shift in our thinking away from the individualising and pathologising of mental disturbance, towards the effects of social and cultural conditions on the daily lives of those most disadvantaged by them. Talwar's book is written by authors who are feminists of colour, those with disabilities and those belonging to LGBTQ+ communities, and is about art therapy with these communities. It is these groups, Talwar says, whose issues have been written out of dominant art therapy discourses, that are at the vanguard of challenging mainstream frameworks of art therapy.

It takes those who have lived it, like the authors in Talwar's book, to see more clearly the everyday racisms and sexist racisms suffered by the marginalised. We, the editors of this book, are both white, middle class and one male, and are therefore more likely to not see, and thus to have a tendency towards unconsciously repeating discrimination or domination in our art therapy work. Although not all our chosen authors were white, the majority are. We began to think that our particular contribution might be to focus the book on how hegemonic power relations of class, race and gender emerge within the clinical work, and how art therapists recognise and work through them. As first drafts were coming in, we directed authors to consider this.

Similarly to Talwar's book, the work in this book comes from one multicultural city, London, UK (with one chapter on a project in Greece with London-based therapists). London, as a centre of financial and political power, can be seen as a microcosm of a global system of social division, inequality and distant and unaccountable elites. This specificity of place allows for a shared context to the chapters in each of the books, revealing more clearly differences in the contrasting cities/countries and their traditions – social action therapy and art therapy for social justice in the US, which Talwar describes, and psychodynamically based art therapy in the UK. The histories we describe are centred from the UK. We would want to avoid any idea of national identities, but specificity of time and place allows for contrast to be seen, compared and learned from.

In addition to Talwar and colleagues, we would position this book, overall, in a relationship to Diane Waller's paradoxical suggestion that UK art therapists are 'pragmatic rebels' (2004). Waller is referring firstly to the contradictions between artists who value the unpredictable and uncanny nature of creativity and free expression and those who wish to fit art into a mental health agenda; and secondly, those who are critics of the establishment but wanting to be accepted as a profession by that establishment. Waller made this suggestion at a time when public services had opportunities for growth and creativity and more capacity to reach marginalised people. In the 19 years since, we have had a ratcheting up of neoliberalism, most forcefully felt through austerity, during which time the health service and welfare services have been further marketised – with private companies awarded contracts often under the banner of 'the NHS'. This fragmentation of the public sector makes the situation for pragmatic rebels very different, though the contradictions remain. Art therapists additionally face the conflicts involved with implementing psychodynamic art therapy practice within institutions that follow establishment agendas such as measurement and targets. The issue of pragmatic rebels, then, is pertinent to the group material. Finally, the argument of this book builds on Chris Wood's (1999, 2011, 2013) almost sole endeavour in art therapy, to discuss class as a relational matter.

COMMUNITY

Art therapy has its roots in a time more favourable than now to communal and collective ways of understanding mental distress and delivering therapy. The NHS and welfare state had been implemented after the second world war in recognition of the fact that the wellbeing of society rested on the health and welfare of all individuals, and therefore it should be collectively paid for through taxation. The art studios of the old asylums, psychiatric day hospitals and therapeutic communities provided art therapy groups that enabled patients to find agency through art making and a sense of belonging to community. This all changed when Margaret Thatcher became prime minister of the UK in 1979.

Thatcher famously said in an interview with the magazine *Woman's Own*, 'there is no such thing as society only individuals and families'. This individualistic ideology, which was paralleled in the US with Ronald Reagan, and soon all over the world, was used to enable the turn towards the privatisation of public services and financialisation – the making of money from money – and the destruction of oppositional communities. The defeat of the miners' strike, through violence, was a critical moment; it allowed the government to seriously curb the power of the unions and to close down most of Britain's manufacturing industries, leading to high unemployment and the break-up of strong communities that had held together for decades. The Labour Party MP, Jon Trickett, in a recent interview (Savage, 2021), describes the effects of this decision on workers in the North of England. Hitherto one or two industries employed thousands of people who then belonged to the same unions and shared a supportive, communal social life based around them. Closing down manufacturing left people without economic purpose and with 'a loss of agency: the belief in the capacity of human beings to collectively act on their environment, to change it, and to impose their will on it'.

The asylums, day hospitals and therapeutic communities were closed down around this time. The policy was termed as moving 'care into the community', and its espoused aim was to relieve the stigma and disempowerment attached to mental illness. However, communities had already been destroyed and patients were left isolated with little support in the context of ever shrinking resources. From this period the 'public' sector workplace began to change, and since the financial crisis of 2008, this change has speeded up.

AUSTERITY

The hostile environment of austerity that the UK has been suffering for more than a decade was a result of the banking crisis in 2008, when the process of rentierism, the making of money out of the investment of profits that had been deregulated in the 1980s, went out of control. Financial institutions across the world had been relying on profits from the mortgages on ever increasing property prices in the USA, and when the housing market bubble burst, they were all bankrupt. Governments, which had been rolled back, were now called on to sort it out, which they did by rescuing the banks, even at the cost of amplifying the recession caused by the sudden credit squeeze, making us all pay for it through austerity measures. The effects of austerity in the UK have been devastating for many. A freedom of information request, to which 50 hospital trusts in England responded (Brewis, 2020), showed that 2,483 children were admitted to hospital with malnutrition between January and June 2020. In December 2020, Unicef, who support children following catastrophes, for the first time in its 70-year history was providing food to malnourished children in the UK, the sixth most wealthy country in the world. Recent research (Redman and Fletcher, 2021) can now show evidence of what was known about the Department of Work and Pensions – that Universal Credit has been a means of making people made vulnerable by the system responsible for their hardship and punishing them for it, leaving the unemployed, the poorly employed, those on low wages and the disabled without money for weeks; many have died as a result. Meanwhile, the housing crisis, brought about by the increased selling off of social housing and more private renting with no rent controls and easy evictions, has led to large numbers of homeless and the breaking up of communities, the effects of these being increasing alienation and mental illness.

People have had to claim benefits and use food banks because the world of work has changed. More and more people are on zero-hour contracts, not knowing if they will get work that day, many have to do two or three or more jobs, whilst others are obliged to commit to one employer only. This has a terrible effect on people – precarious work never ends, the worker must always be available with no claims to a private life; there are always others to take your place as now what is bought is packages of time, not the work of an individual. Nowadays almost all forms of work are precarious. Meanwhile, there is yet a further underclass; Britain's and the USA's imperialist wars have led to large numbers of displaced persons needing sanctuary in the UK but not actually getting it. Migrant and immigrant populations are treated as a sub-class, amongst whom political insecurity, lack of full citizenship rights and racism enable employers to exploit them even more ruthlessly in modern forms akin to slavery.

Art therapists' work has progressively become more precarious with increases in temporary contracts, sessional employment, honorary contracts and voluntary positions (MacKinnon et al., 2017). Alarmingly, 14.65% of respondents to a British Association of Art Therapists (BAAT) survey (BAAT, 2018) had no contract.

MARGINALISATION

Naomi Klein's 'disaster capitalism' (2007) describes how displaced persons from wars and tragedies are being treated as a valuable commodity in the market. A whole private financial industry exists around refugee camps, detention centres, prisons, enforcement agencies and so on. We are accustomed to think of wars as between countries, but it appears that the purpose of wars is to feed, not only the arms industry, but now these other companies like Serco and G4S. We see that the distress of the people with whom we work is not only the result of an uncaring system – the creation and exploitation of distress has been a political choice that has enabled capitalism to reinvent itself and carry on.

We, art therapists, have prided ourselves on our work with these marginalised groups in the public sector, and now in charities and other organisations, when traditionally other therapists have been more likely to work with those able to pay (Waller, 1991, Wood, 1999). It is reassuring to see that in response to the Black Lives Matter movement, BAAT, in consultation with the membership, has devised a statement which acknowledges the systemic nature of racist oppression (BAAT, 2020). We think, though, that it is essential that structural racism and oppression are recognised as written into the neoliberal agenda. Until this link is made, and we can comprehend the enormous limitations we face in helping those most affected by the system, very little progress can be made. James Baldwin, in the film, 'I am not your negro', asks, 'Why do white people need the negro?' (Peck, 2016). This question raises the issue of white people's complicity in the necessity of a 'denigrated' (the Latin origin of the word, lowered by being black) 'other' for the maintenance of capitalism.

In the same statement, BAAT says that art therapists have used the arts to help clients to find their own unique mark, and to express something of their experience, in their own way. Whilst a recognition of individuality is an important means of valuing those who are marginalised, the emphasis on the individual contributes to an idea that art therapy can treat the effects of racism. As Gipson (2017) says, it 'distances professional ethics from wider historical issues of power ... well-meaning professional caregivers participate in the process of disconnecting interpersonal experiences from political and economic forces that affect everyday human life' (p116). The fact that a current day map of the most impoverished peoples would map straight onto a map of black and brown skinned people tells us all we need to know about the legacy and on-going practices of colonialism, and what has to be done to confront the problems of structural racism. It is disappointing in this light to read that BAAT, in the same statement (BAAT 2020), declares itself to be a non-political organisation.

Around 90% of the art therapy profession are women and the implications of this are of interest. It is an essential feature of capitalism that 'unproductive' work, in the form of the care needed to maintain a workforce that labours to produce, is done unpaid. Hence women have been the ones to raise the children, keep the home, care for the sick and elderly, all without remuneration. Where they are employed in paid work it is usually in the care sector and thus low waged. It is important that we recognise that endemic discrimination in class, race and gender, as well as in disability, religion, sexuality, age and so on, combined in their various groupings in the term 'intersectionality', all stem from the same cause – the domination of the working class through violence or the threat of violence.

Art therapists working in the care sector are, on the whole, alert to the political context of our work, it often appears more so than some other healthcare practitioners who are arguably more protected by recognised status. However, neoliberalism works in a way that draws us in to perform in ways that collude with the interests of the few and against the interests of the many without us often being conscious of it.

Due to therapy's origins within colonialism, therapists have inherited much of the authority and certainty that white colonialists have had in relation to 'others'; we have seen ourselves as at the centre of an understanding of the human condition, the creators and authors of history, the discoverers of the rest of the world (Blackwell, 2003). These colonial patterns of relationship, Blackwell argues, remain deep in our social unconscious and the significance of skin colour is embedded in our psyches. This has fitted into social class structure, with upper and middle classes concerned with the maintenance of superiority and social difference. Non-whites become more acceptable as they adopt white, middle-class values. Hostility is replaced by paternalism, condescension, conditional acceptance, tolerance and kindness rather than respect as equals. Our heritage as art therapists, then, is the missionary, helping the poor African children by diverting them from their 'primitive ways' and teaching them the values of Christian religion.

CONCLUSION

There is a temptation for art therapists, for all therapists, to deal with the immense suffering brought about by neoliberalism by separating ourselves from it – seeing it only in our clients who we can then feel good about helping. For art therapists, the agency in art making and the empowerment that can be felt from that can seem like tools we have that counter the hostile environment. However, this position of helper and helped can lead us to unknowingly replicate unequal power relations within the therapy and, paradoxically, disempower our clients. It is not possible to separate art therapy from the political systems of domination in which it exists, but in recognising the ways in which they invade our art therapy groups, we can become aware of the dynamics of collusion or resistance, or to use Waller's words, pragmatism or rebellion.

The next chapter looks further into the way the privatisation for profit agenda of neoliberalism has invaded our institutions, presenting contradictions between our own intentions for art therapy and those of the profiteers, whose interests are becoming increasingly embedded in all of our institutional structures, and thus the priorities of our managers. We explore how neoliberal priorities invade our own thinking as we attempt to be pragmatic and maintain an art therapy service in antithetical conditions.

REFERENCES

BAAT (2018). *BAAT Workforce Survey 2018.*

BAAT (2020). *Increasing Equality, Diversity and Inclusion in Art Therapy CRM:0003689.* [PDF] London: BAAT.

Blackwell, D. (2003). Colonialism and globalization: A group-analytic perspective. *Group Analysis*, 27th S.H. Foulkes Annual Lecture, 36(4), pp. 445–463.

Brewis, H. (2020). 'Nearly 2,500 children hospitalised with malnutrition since January, new research shows'. *Evening Standard*, 12th July. Available at: https://www.standard.co.uk/news/uk/2-500-children-hospitalised-malnutrition-england-a4496106.html [Accessed 29th June 2021].

de Maré, P.B., Piper, R., Thompson, S. (1991). *Koinonia: From Hate, Through Dialogue, to Culture in the Large Group.* London: Karnac Books.

Fisher, M. (2012). 'Why mental health is a political issue'. *The Guardian*, 16th July [online]. Available at: https://www.theguardian.com/commentisfree/2012/jul/16/mental-health-political-issue [Accessed 29th June 2021].

Gipson, L. (2017). Challenging neoliberalism and multicultural love in art therapy. *Art Therapy*, 34(3), pp.112–117.

Hogan, S. (2015). *Art Therapy Theories: A Critical Introduction.* 1st ed., London: Routledge.

Klein, N. (2007). *The Shock Doctrine: The Rise of Disaster Capitalism*. London and New York: Macmillan.

MacKinnon, E., Myles, A., Page, K., Shelhi, T. and Westwood, J. (2017). Shifting terrains: Art psychotherapists' testimonies and reflections on employment in austerity Britain. *Art Therapy OnLine*, 8(2), pp.1–34.

Peck, R. [director] (2016) *I am not your Negro* [film].

Redman, J. and Fletcher, D.R. (2021). Violent bureaucracy: A critical analysis of the British public employment service. *Critical Social Policy*. https://doi.org/10.1177/02610183211001766

Savage, L. (2021). 'Labour must fight a class war, not a culture war. An interview with Jon Trickett'. *Jacobin*, 15th March. Available at: https://www.jacobinmag.com/2021/03/jon-trickett-interview-class-war-culture-war-labour-party-deindustrialization [Accessed on 29th June 2021].

Skaife, S. (2001). Making visible: Art therapy and intersubjectivity. *International Journal of Art Therapy: Inscape*, 6(2), pp. 40–50.

Skaife, S. (2013). Black and White: Applying Derrida to contradictory experiences in an art therapy group for victims of torture. *Group Analysis*, 46(3), pp. 256–271.

Skaife, S., Morris, L., Tipple, R. and Velada, D. (2020). The story of the camera, a case study of an art therapy large group. *Group Analysis*, 53(1), pp. 37–59.

Springham, N., Findlay, D., Woods, A. and Harris, J. (2012). How can art therapy contribute to mentalization in borderline personality disorder? *International Journal of Art Therapy*, 17(3), pp. 115–129.

Talwar, S.K. (ed.) (2018). *Art Therapy for Social Justice: Radical Intersections*. 1st ed., New York and London: Routledge.

Waller, D. (1991). *Becoming a Profession (Psychology Revivals): The History of Art Therapy in Britain 1940–82*. London and New York: Routledge.

Waller, D. (2004). *Art Therapists: Pragmatic Rebels*. London: Goldsmiths College, University of London.

Wood, C. (1999). Class Issues in Therapy. In: Campbell, J. (ed.), *Art therapy, Race and Culture*. London and Philadelphia: Jessica Kingsley Publishers, pp. 135–156.

Wood, C. (2011). The Evolution of Art Therapy in Relation to Psychosis and Poverty. In: Gilroy, A. (ed.), *Art Therapy Research in Practice*. Bern: Peter Lang, pp. 211–229.

Wood, C. (ed.) (2013). *Navigating Art Therapy: A Therapist's Companion*. London and New York: Routledge.

CHAPTER TWO

Caught in contradiction

Sally Skaife and Jon Martyn

DOI: 10.4324/9781003107408-3

INTRODUCTION

In this chapter we look at the contradictions that have arisen in institutions in which art therapy is involved that have resulted from the ideology of neoliberalism. An NHS setting, a university art therapy training setting and our professional association, the British Association of Art Therapists (BAAT), are seen to have been impacted in some similar ways. We consider how a likely internalisation of neoliberalist values can lead us to replicate these in our practices.

We argue, in the tradition of many others before us, from de Boettie (1577) to Fisher (2012), that capitalism only continues because of our complicity, and that to counteract this we need to be aware of our role in maintaining the system and to take creative control of its inherent contradictions.

We consider two central contradictions that have followed the privatisation of public services, the first is the focus on individualism whilst simultaneously individuals are neglected, and the second is the privileging of disembodied rationality despite art therapy involving the specificity of materiality in art and complex social relationships.

AN NHS WORKPLACE

An art therapist writes:

In 2010 I joined an organisation, 'The Retreat', a former residential therapeutic community, which had been reformed to become a personality disorder outpatient service. The service retained elements of the therapeutic community, providing non-residential treatment to people who were able to self-refer without the need for diagnosis. With the emphasis still on group work and patient-led social spaces, the aims were building trusting relationships, where this was a serious area of difficulty, and fostering a sense of individual and collective responsibility. Patients developed a relationship with the service, the building and the practitioners, the majority of whom had been in the service for over a decade.

Some months after I had begun work there, a problem arose with the location of the service, which was away from the centre and thus seen as limiting patient access. Trust funding was acquired to establish an outreach group, and a number of suitable, unused buildings within the trust's hospital grounds were identified. The only problem was that the trust's newly established 'internal market' meant that the service would need to pay the trust's central office to hire these buildings. The community group was not funded to pay for rental costs and the trust was not willing to waive the hire fee, so that was that. A madness, as this was money which would have been cost neutral either way.

Thanks to national policy focused on shortening waiting lists, the trust was also under constant threat of being fined, then £300 per patient waiting to be seen for more than eighteen weeks. The trust was placing pressure on the service for its long waiting lists, as if it was to blame for the high levels of social distress and the resultant demand for specialist long-term treatment. The service was forced to create a solution to this problem and began to offer group assessment sessions where a group of up to thirty referrals would be invited to the service for a half day introduction. From a management perspective this was a great innovation; the service was able to reduce the waiting list and meet with a huge volume of referrals using only a few members of staff. However, this large group experience would often be overwhelming, leaving fragile patients to disengage. Less demand for the service meant less scrutiny from the trust management as the trust faced fewer government fines. I was aware of this system being a deterrent, but I marvelled at the ingenuity afoot and agreed with the rationale that disengaged patients, in any case, were not going to be suitable for group therapy.

The service, though highly respected, was also seen as costly and inefficient due to the complexity and length of treatment programmes. Whilst the organisation was acting as a preventative measure keeping patients out of crisis care, this cost was not included in budget calculations as it was recorded in a separate budget in a separate service. The service manager, knowing that good work was done, would frequently complain that we were not providing adequate evidence of our work. There was an expectation that

*we would gather CORE forms (Clinical Outcomes in Routine Evaluation –
a self-rated questionnaire which measures psychological problems and
distress). We were warned of the consequences of non-compliance and were
monitored to ensure we did the job. Yet these forms were never analysed.
They sat untouched, growing in mass, in a filing cabinet; no one in the team
had capacity, training or motivation to analyse them. When the service
manager raised this with his managers, he was told that the trust was not
willing to employ someone to scrutinise this data, nor was anyone permitted
to reduce their patient contact time to attend to this growing bulk. We were
all stuck in a bind – patients would frequently complain of the intrusive
nature of the questions while staff members were expected to hurriedly
collect the data in the knowledge that forms would just be left to gather dust.*

*This was the early years of austerity and the service was implementing
cuts actually devised under the Labour government. There was a growing
sense of mistrust – a belief that the cuts would be poorly implemented. The
service manager – a white 'well-spoken' man – became a focus for staff and
patient discontent. In a team meeting the topic of performance review was
being discussed. One staff member was dismayed about cuts to the training
budget; these performance reviews were meaningless if staff development
was not being supported. Discussion became heated. The service
manager became exasperated and shared his recent experience of his own
performance review. He explained that his own line manager had written it
before they had met and he was expected to sign it without discussion. He
was indicating that his role was to 'manage' and implement decisions which
had been made by his superiors. This disclosure punctured our collective
illusion of his potency and yet revealed something more difficult – the
service manager was not destroying the service nor was he able to save it. In
essence, we were all powerless together.*

*The service was forced to reform in 2012; self-referrals were no longer
permitted and new patients needed a personality disorder diagnosis or their
treatment would not be funded. The trust sold the building and grounds to
a housing developer and the service was renamed, with its link to its history
and sense of community removed, replaced by a purely diagnostic title,
Personality Disorder Treatment Service. The service was relocated to the*

city's hospital groups, with treatment programmes and posts cut, including one of two art therapy posts.

This hospital service is a powerful example of the contradictions that arise when a public sector service that aims to help is run as a business whose aim is profit. The internal market in the trust meant that to respond to the needs of the community for better access, money had to be spent on hiring an unused building the trust already owned; here the philosophy of profit making had not only resulted in less benefit for the clients, it was in direct contradiction with the aim for efficiency itself. Another absurd contradiction was that the service was punished with fines for its high demand; in a true marketplace a business with a long waiting list would expand and provide more treatment instead of having impediments put in its way.

The business philosophy actually spelled the demise of this successful service as a recognisable therapeutic community; not simply through cuts and closure but by infiltrating and undermining the ethos of community as treatment. The dignity and ownership that went along with self-referral, and the emphasis on mutual relationship, was replaced by the creation of 'service users', a name that differentiates them from 'service providers'. The 'service' suggests that the priority is one of processing them as if they are the sum of their file. People in distress were processed into patients-with-diagnoses, but then these same people/commodities were also the consumers of our other product, packages-of-treatment, in our case, 'art therapy'. As consumers, service users rate the treatment product through CORE forms. These CORE forms were not only found by patients to be intrusive and by staff to feel pointless, as the data gained remained unused, but the individualised questions about symptoms presented a contradiction to a service which was about interdependence and the encouragement of patient responsibility. The idea that all outcomes are measurable is absurd and the pressure on patients to comply with this notion is a further attack on dignity and on the value of the relationships they formed. This mismatch shows why therapeutic communities, as they were originally conceived, have all but vanished.

The waiting list problem was solved unethically, however the head of the service was not responsible – the problem had been handed down, the manager on site was not responsible – just following the targets, and the therapists were just doing what they were told. Dalal (2018) argues that the increase in hierarchy in organisations is related to the knowledge that cuts do harm and that no one wants to be directly responsible for it.

In this NHS example we see a number of contradictions that have resulted from the invasion of the market into the workplace. The trust scores 'own goals' as the profit principle has not resulted in the efficiency it desires; staff are neither able to do the job as they wish, nor are they able to do what the service is now requiring as there is insufficient time for bureaucracy; clients are individualised in a service that addresses interpersonal relationships; and those most in need of the service become excluded from it through the system of assessment, and are made to feel it is because of their own inadequacies.

The introduction of the profit motive into another public institution employing art therapists – the university – whose goal is education and research, shows similar contradictions and own goals, such as inefficiency and the inhibition of a learning culture.

IN A UNIVERSITY

An art therapy educator writes:

There was a point at which I suddenly discovered that my job had changed and that I ought to have known it already, though it was never spelled out. My energies were now to be redirected to bringing increased income into the university and networking in search of opportunities. Already, our time to teach the art therapy programme had been gradually whittled down by increasing bureaucracy – filling in time management sheets, research output forms – several different ones for different purposes, self-evaluation, programme evaluation, evaluation of evaluation, giving words to every facet of the art therapy training to match against criteria for quality assurance inside and outside the university. Our admin staff who had previously worked closely with us and understood the work well enough to support it independently now were told that they weren't paid to think but only to follow our instructions. This led to numerous unnecessary misunderstandings and extra work for all.

There was some sharing in the department as a whole of the new situation that faced us, that is, that we were all having to conform to a government agenda which had set universities in competition, with inadequate resources, and that the survival of us all depended on us becoming entrepreneurs. We were in it together. However, it took on a personal, bullying tone. It was made clear that unless you met research targets or became a manager yourself, you were only of minor use and, as was once said by a manager, 'dead wood'. This attitude to staff was mirrored in that towards students, with quite punitive protocols over assessment, for example.

We were encouraged to regard the art therapy training as akin to other non-therapy vocational training and for it to be run similarly, preferably with joint teaching. Our interest in our subject and the quality of the programme were seen in a negative way, we were frequently told that we were 'siloed', stuck in the past, and should not think of ourselves as special. The way budgets were managed resulted in the programme usually being in debt despite high recruitment; we were told that its costs were being covered by other programmes to their detriment and that we were responsible.

The worst of it was, though, that I would catch myself operating with some of the same, dominant values. I wanted to succeed within the criteria of the university and I also wanted to do whatever it took for the university to survive and flourish as I identified with it. I felt I had been swallowed up in a poisonous system that I recognised as such but could not see the way out of.

It was on the picket line during a trade union backed dispute with management over pensions being cut that I discovered that staff in other departments were having similar experiences and had ideas for making the university a more democratic place. This gave us all some strength.

This art therapist educator's experience of the exponential increase in bureaucracy is widespread everywhere. Ironically, the argument for bringing the market into public services was that the private sector did well because competition reduced bureaucracy, yet we have seen a massive increase in bureaucracy in public services (Dalal, 2016). Prior to the privatisation of the NHS, just 4% of the overall budget was spent on admin, now it is 12–15% (Gill, 2019). All this bureaucracy has created the need for managerialism to ensure that it is done in the required way; at the base of which is the notion that workers are not to be trusted. What operates is 'a culture that is highly regulated, highly controlled, very rigid, and often very punitive' (Dalal, 2018, p. 88). The aim is control of the workforce through the creation of multiple protocols and procedures, and the micromanagement of checking performance in relation to targets and adjusting rewards accordingly. In order not to overwork managers, more and more of the surveillance is given to workers themselves who end up in a constant state of anxiety about their readiness for the next appraisal. Fisher (2009) echoes Foucault in pointing out that in bureaucratised institutions it isn't necessary for all the staff to be surveilled all the time, since the surveillance is internalised. Time spent on bureaucracy is time spent away from the main task, education and research, and is therefore antithetical to the university's purpose.

Dalal (2016) talks of how public services are required to show value for money but do this by using the methods applicable to the mechanics of manufacturing, which come unstuck when used for people. Yet measurement has become the rule of the day, the quantification of everything with the detachment of numbers can mean that no one is responsible. Audit and protocols are without authors so they cannot be critiqued; neither can they be applied flexibly, as they would if they did have an author. Admin staff being told their job was not to think removes any meaningfulness from work. Performance, that is, the practice of art therapy or teaching, is not easily quantifiable, so it needs more and more audits which end up bearing little relation to actual practice. All this enables services to be packaged and reproduced, losing their connection to history, place or people.

Public relations representations have become everything; a university is known by its rating for research via the Research Excellence

Framework (REF) and teaching by the Teaching Excellence Framework (TEF); schools are measured by OFSTED (Office for Standards in Education), and hospitals by National Institute for Health and Care Excellence (NICE)-approved treatments. The competition engendered by ratings means that they are inevitably massaged and manipulated. These targets are supposed to be about ensuring best practice but actually are a means of giving parents and patients the idea that they have a choice. Choice is an illusion of empowerment since the choices are, by definition, limited – not all of the children can go to the 'best' school – whilst offering choice opens doors to privatisation of more and more services.

The art therapist and the educator speak of being sucked into the system and this again seems part of how the apparatus now functions. Dalal (2016) talks of how our human need for recognition, for value and acceptance get manipulated. For example, the 'employee of the year' encourages us to compete with one another. Managers may have taken on the role with a genuine belief that they would prioritise their responsibility towards staff over that of the efficiency drive of the institution. However they are caught, flattered or threatened in some way into taking on the role, they will only survive by following the dictates of their own managers and exercising power over those below them in the hierarchy. As Fisher eloquently writes,

> watch someone step up into management and it's usually not very long before the grey petrification of power starts to subsume them. It is here that structure is palpable – you can practically see it taking people over, hear its deadened/deadening judgements speaking through them.
>
> (Fisher, 2012, p. 69)

The increase in competition, bureaucracy, audit and protocols, as well as hierarchy, that we have described in our workplaces can be seen operating within our professional association, BAAT.

A PROFESSIONAL ASSOCIATION

During most of its existence BAAT has either been working towards, or within, the government body now called the Health and Care Professions Council (HCPC). The intention was to achieve a secure place for art therapy in public provision and to protect standards. Prior to this, many art therapists had been pushed here and there in ad hoc positions, often employed in other roles such as adult art educators and had been unable to offer any consistent therapy; anybody could call themselves art therapists regardless of training, but now regulation would protect the title and, in doing so, protect the public. When state regulation was eventually established in 1997, a question was posed about the role of BAAT as it would no longer be the regulator of training nor of professional standards, roles now taken by the Health Professions Council (HPC) as it was then called. It would instead have an advisory function to HPC, alongside the training establishments and that of individual art therapists.

BAAT's response was to set itself up in competition with the university-based training courses. Continuing Professional Development (CPD) courses and introductory courses, which had previously been run in the universities, were now offered by BAAT at a cheaper rate. Universities and other sources of training were charged (and continue to be at the time of writing) large sums of money by BAAT to advertise their non-qualifying courses through the only mailing list of art therapists available. BAAT has, in recent years, aligned itself with the company PG Mutual for special reductions for consumer purchases on the high street, gym membership, entry to golf courses and more. It seems that BAAT has been moving away from being an association of its members to behaving like a small business, part-funded by membership subscriptions, which monopolises the CPD market. There is a confusion over whether BAAT members are the products or the consumers of BAAT produced CPD. This creates contradictions for members whereby some are unable to use the association for support in their work in the form of advertising it, and some will not be able to access non-BAAT CPD because they will not hear about it, that is, if it is possible for it to be put on at all. At one time it was a prerequisite of BAAT membership that members belonged to a trade union. On a BAAT survey in 2019, however, only 43.5% were in a union, which reflects its change in direction.

Since 2019 BAAT has become a Company. Council, renamed the Board of Directors, are the body legally responsible for the organisation and so make the decisions. Thus, proposals made at AGMs are no longer binding on Council. In line with this the association appears to have become increasingly hierarchical and undemocratic. From the top down there is the CEO, now a job-share, then the Board of Directors, then parallel Regional Coordinators, Special Interest Group co-ordinators (SIGs) and an Art Therapy Practice Network co-ordinator, who are all accountable to the Directors. One of the current job-share CEOs, whose only work experience of therapy is as a CEO, has the following job description: 'To provide leadership and clear strategic direction for the development and management of BAAT so that it is recognised as a beacon of dynamism and innovation for UK art therapy'. In a democratic organisation the person providing leadership and direction should be elected by the members. The coordinators of the SIG groups seem to be in a middle management role, they are expected to give direction and leadership and to ensure that the aims and approach of the SIG are maintained in accordance with the Board of Directors. Minutes of meetings must be sent to the unelected CEO. All groups have quite specific aims that have been devised by BAAT, in particular, research is meant to be at the heart of all of them, with different aspects of research specifically outlined. BAAT has created detailed Standards of Practice on top of the HCPC ones; those for private practitioners include questions to ask at assessment to all clients regardless of race, gender and so on to be in line with equal opportunities, suggesting art therapy is something to be formulaically applied.

BAAT internal correspondence has revealed that criticisms of the Board of Directors or CEOs have often been met with intimidating and threatening responses. On one of the members' forums there is a threat that if members post anything that the Board of Directors perceives as unsuitable they may be referred to the HCPC under 'fitness to practice'. There seems to be a preoccupation with risk and harm, though in actuality the number of arts therapists that have been struck off by HCPC is only 0.16% of members of all art therapies professions, and only 16 cases out of the 77 referred were seen to merit pursuit (Springham and Huet, 2020). There is a danger that harmful behaviour is getting located in individual practitioners rather than in the system. We can see from the institutional examples above that harm is embedded in the apparatus itself, and an emphasis on individuals can both mask and collude with this. The managerialism that Dalal (2018) refers to as necessary because workers are not to be trusted seems applicable here. BAAT members are not to be trusted – indeed, to make it onto the private practitioners' list, art therapists have to produce descriptions of case work in a prescribed form for vetting on criteria that are not made transparent.

It is now often the case that managers are no longer professionals of the service they manage and know little about the actual job they are managing, as is the case with the job-share CEO. This is not seen to matter because it is the system, known by its representations, that is prioritised and the system can be transported. The result of this is manualisation – the idea is that the organisation and the work it does can be fully known in advance, delivered and measured (Dalal, 2018). There is a clear similarity here with the development of models of art therapy.

Where art therapy has valued interpersonal relationships as the context of treatment, neoliberalism throws up the individual-with-a-lack to be processed and measured; where art therapy has valued play with an unknown outcome, neoliberalism throws up hyper-rationality and manualisaton, also to be measured. The result is a loss of meaningfulness and a lack of soul.

Unsurprisingly, art therapists can end up internalising priorities that run counter to its basic values, suppressing the contradictions.

INDIVIDUALISM/VALUING THE INDIVIDUAL

The individualising ideology of neoliberalism has been highly successful, permeating its way into all aspects of life, and thus, art therapy. For example, though groups can be the form of treatment in contemporary art therapy, the energy and money is put into assessment and measurement of individuals, rather than into the supportive infrastructure that bolsters up the collective, the building and the staff team that can enable the community as a whole to do the work. Lost are the art studios which enabled patients to discover agency in art making and a sense of belonging. Also lost to the margins is the original sense of the therapy group, as group reflection of the group by the group and for the group, including the staff – adapted from Foulkes and Anthony (1965).

Whilst capitalism favours individualism over community, it paradoxically devalues individuals' experience. As a system reliant on inequality, capitalism has normalised a lack of care as necessary collateral damage. The richest, who are most dependent on care, employing nannies, cleaners and so on, are able to deny their need for care by projecting their dependency onto those they make dependent through paying paltry wages for their caring work. Meanwhile, those needing care from public services are denounced and humiliated (Hakim et al., 2020).

Frances Walton (2016) describes the systematic and exponential way in which the government has withdrawn from a responsibility for those with mental distress, replacing 'dependency' with Personal Health Budgets (PhB) that allow patients to become 'experts in their own recovery'. PhBs allow them to purchase short stints of NICE-approved therapy, usually cognitive behavioural therapy (CBT), art classes and gym membership, for example – activities which are not about building relationships. In her reflections, Walton balances the loss of personal attachments to buildings, teams and therapists with the benefits of independence and personal choice, paralleling her own move from a reliance on the workplace to working privately and 'managing' herself.

In another paper on adult mental health, Rothwell and Grandison (2016) draw on Fuller's (2013) psychic stages of recovery for their art therapy plan for service users moving from acute to community settings: 'a lack of a consistent cohesive sense of self during an acute admission' (undifferentiated sense of self), 'an emerging sense of self, through to a more stable sense of self (differentiated)' (Rothwell and Grandison,

2016, p. 181). The language is entirely individual, though the treatment is actually in groups. The aim is for 'social recovery' and the 'care pathway to recovery' is described as 'patient led'.

There is something disingenuous in these terms used in adult mental health. It seems unlikely that patients experiencing psychosis or severe depression are going to easily manage PhBs, however attractive the notion of being 'experts', getting 'care' and achieving 'recovery' sound. That failure will be felt as their personal failure. Rothwell and Grandison (2016) describe their plan as something to be kept in mind, as patients are frequently readmitted, sometimes involuntarily, and circumstances change. The reality, as one would expect in the hostile environment, appears to be much messier than what is suggested by 'care pathways to recovery'. The idea that the plan is 'patient led' seems to be contradicted by a system that relies on dominant white discourses of recovery, not differentiating between social or racial background. In both these articles the art therapists stress the need for therapists' adaptation to, and flexibility with, the limits of the system. Despite both the chapters discussing support in the community, what seems assumed by the service and the art therapists is that independence is a desirable goal. It is interesting to note that in BAAT's description of art therapy (BAAT, 2021) there is no mention of the therapeutic relationship, as if the therapist is an invisible provider of art therapy methods.

Val Huet (2012) writes about creativity in a 'cold climate'. She explores the devaluation of work in a pilot research project in which a group of middle management NHS nurses make art in response to looking at art on the hospital walls, and in the process, tell moving stories about their working life. One nurse speaks of the way that the organisation has ridiculed their day-to-day hard work, completely undermining and devaluing it. Huet speaks of the staff's stress, isolation, fatigue and helplessness, and talks of a freezing and paralysis of creativity. Huet's paper argues that staff in organisations can cultivate their creativity through art therapy, enabling a freeing of imagination. This has seemed to be the case in this example. However, unless we take this a step further and link the benefits that come from creativity to collective benefits, which might enable resistance and foster imagination of how different the world could be without capitalism, there is a danger of the outcome sounding like an entrepreneurial promotion of our product for soothing the effects of an inhumane system, and so propping it up.

The idea of therapy as the solution to our unhappiness has been crucial for the success of neoliberalism (Fisher, 2012). It is linked to the propagation of self-help doctrines, both in therapy treatment (such as CBT) and in popular culture, such as self-help television shows and self-help books. Smail (2005) calls this tendency 'magical voluntarism', the idea that the therapist can magically cure the patient of their distress with their rituals and potions, for example, with our interpretations. Art therapists' potions might nowadays be 'evidence-based' interventions. Smail suggests that therapists are invested in this idea not only because their livelihoods depend on it, but also their self-worth and status; however, this self-interest goes unacknowledged. It is complicated as patients, too, are invested in magical voluntarism – we all like the idea of magic. The art therapist Gipson (2017, p. 112) describes disavowal of self-interest as perpetuating a situation in which art therapists can imagine we are 'outside of the social world that produces the issues that bring people to counseling'. The whole therapy project requires us to project our own feelings of dehumanisation, lack of being valued and need for attention onto 'the other' who we help. We see something of this happening in the recent emphasis on service user representation.

The service user movement and 'dual experience' (referring to those who have been, or are, both patients within the psychiatric services and professional art therapists) expertise have taken a front seat in art therapy in recent years (Morgan et al., 2012, Woods and Springham, 2012, Huet and Holttum, 2016, Wood, 2020), perhaps due to the HCPC embedding consultation with service users and carers in its Standards for Education (HCPC, 2014). On the one hand, this looks like the 'patient', who traditionally has very little power in psychiatric services, being given or taking power, and thus seems like a form of resistance to the stigmatisation of mental illness. However, it seems to also stem from, and lead back to, an individualised way of understanding distress.

The service user movement has been around for about 40 years, yet, as a concept, it has never been completely clear what it is (Millar et al., 2016). Millar's concept analysis produced five key attributes – person-centred approach, informed decision making, advocacy, obtaining service users' views and feedback. Most art therapy papers seem to relate to the first and maybe last categories.

It is upsetting to read under Millar's 'person-centred' category that service users in mental health need to advise mental health workers of the importance of their being listened to, of receiving empathy, attempts to understand them, respect and dignity. Art therapist service users' accounts of their experience in the literature similarly describe dreadful stigmatisation of mental distress. It is not surprising that a proportion of society should have to carry, for the rest of us, feelings of uselessness, anxiety, fear and so on. This projection and 'othering' is necessary for the maintenance of the go-getting, positivist, self-promoting culture that feeds neoliberalism. In promoting the service user voice are we not disavowing our own self-interest, as Gipson (2017) describes?

Huet and Holttum (2016) point to a paradox – that in inviting service users to share their experiences in art therapist education, the idea that they are the ones who have negative experiences is reinforced, increasing stigmatisation. They suggest that this might be resolved by facilitating therapists who themselves have been service users to teach, creating them as experts by experience. The issue with this is that though the service user may have experience that most therapists don't have, that is a mental health diagnosis and experience as an in or out patient, each service user will have different experiences of this. No one individual can speak for all. All of us have experience of mental suffering to different degrees and should be able to empathise with any individual's unique experience. Therapists relate to others' suffering based on in-depth reflection on our own in personal therapy. Therapists need to learn not from individual representatives of service users, but from the person we have in front of us, about how being a service user has affected them. It is important, too, to keep in mind that what happens in the therapy space, and the art made in it, is a co-production. Different art works will be made with different therapists and other group members. A person's difficulties cannot be separated from the particular therapist relating to them or from the positionality of the creators of the so-called objective form they fill in.

This is not to say that the collective activities of service users – such as the Hearing Voices Movement described by Wood (2013, 2020) – are not valuable, far from it. But this is service users working together for goals of their own choosing, rather than individuals being co-opted to the agenda of art therapists (even if that art therapist is themselves) and required to conform to priorities that conflict with service users' interests. Such priorities include the requirement to conform to evidence-based treatment methods acceptable to NICE, which privilege cognitively based therapies.

HYPER-RATIONALITY

Art is material, embodied and takes its meaning from context. In contradiction, what has become valued in art therapy is disembodied practices separated from context. We saw how these appear in BAAT documents in standards of practice and guidelines; they are also embedded in much art therapy research.

When the notion of evidence-based practice was introduced alongside neoliberalism in the 1980s and 1990s fear was expressed about losing everything we most valued about art therapy – the creative and anti-establishment potential in art, for example. Art therapists, though, took a pragmatic approach, embracing audit and guidelines and research. Gilroy's (2006) view was that whilst art therapists should remain alert to the politics involved and to the privileging of 'gold standard' research methods, such as randomised control trials that are not easily implemented in art therapy, we should nevertheless embrace research using a plurality of methods, including finding our own suited to our particular practice. To not do this would be to our peril, and the efforts to find out what worked best for whom could also help to improve practice.

Such pragmatism has not made noticeable gains for us in the mental health marketplace, art therapy losing out to treatments such as CBT, which have the production of outcome measures built into their design. Dalal (2018) compares Improving Access to Psychological Therapies (IAPT) programme's dominance of the mental health sector to an aggressive corporate takeover, where the evidence base has been gamed and corrupted to produce results which gain favour with commissioning bodies in order to further market growth.

Working out what works best for whom, though it sounds laudable, inevitably requires diagnosis, or clusters based on 'needs', and it requires manualised treatment that can be measured. In recent years the profession has embraced mentalisation based therapy (MBT), a treatment method created and manualised by Peter Fonagy and Anthony Bateman for clients with borderline personality disorder (BPD) (Franks and Whitaker, 2007, Or, 2010, Springham et al., 2012, Havsteen-Franklin and Altamirano, 2015, Springham and Camic, 2017). MBT regards the BPD patient as having an impaired capacity to think with affect and to understand others' minds. The therapy aims to increase the thinking capacity and the method is the practice of rationality. Similar to CBT, the treatment appears aligned with the research method and with cost effectiveness in mind. 'This treatment can be implemented by generic mental health professionals with experience of working with personality disorder; only moderate levels of additional training are required' (Bateman and Fonagy, 2013, p. 599).

Springham and Camic's research (2017) on art therapy MBT with BPD service users focuses on 'what good therapists do' and uses grounded theory analysis of observed practice. Sixteen observers in four groups of differently interested people observe video extracts chosen by the art therapists of three groups on the basis of what they think is their best practice in the art looking phase of the group. In line with the method, observations are coded and categorised. The mentalising approach gives quite explicit instructions on how therapists should behave, and the behaviour observations mirror this, appearing quite mechanical, 'art

therapist demonstrating attention', 'art therapist appearing passive' –
all behaviour becoming separated from its field when turned into
prescriptive findings, the main one being that good art therapists working
with BPD individuals actively keep the focus of the group on thinking
about the art in the discussion part of the group, as this enables 'chaotic
and dismissive groups to cooperate' (p. 1).

Tipple (2017) argues that MBT's overemphasis on mental representations
results in it obscuring the relationship between images in groups, group
dynamics and the embodied, material and culturally conditioned aspects
of mind and thinking. As such, it does not engage with the social and
political at all. Based on Springham and Camic's (2017) paper it appears
that the only reason for making art in MBT is for encouraging the artist
and the viewers to mentalise about it. Chaos and defeatism could be
regarded as a necessary part of the creative process, both in art and in
groups, but in MBT it seems that, along with subjectivity, they are to be
tidied up.

Andrew Marshall-Tierney (2014), in a contrasting paper, writes a
powerful personal account of making art alongside his clients on an
acute forensic ward, discussing the paradoxes involved when art is
a joint production between therapist and patients. The art therapy
described shows an alternative way of being with human distress
than those derived from psychiatry and psychology. He says, 'By art
making I hope to show toleration for ambiguity and uncertainty; I
value not-knowing in an environment that tends to foreclose meaning'
(2014, p. 99). This is not a research paper, yet it ends up with a list of
recommendations that he expects to be applicable to other art therapy
situations, which seems to contradict the ambiguity he has spoken
of earlier. The recommendations consist of a list of dos and don'ts
which close meaning down: 'let patients view, handle and modify the
therapist's art work', 'begin art making whether or not patients are in
the room' (2014, p. 105). It is an example of what Dalal (2018) says
about us being steeped in an evidence-based mentality that demands
that the value of any experience is in its capacity to be turned into a set
of actions to be copied.

This dominance of research has led to very particular ways of conceptualising and discussing art therapy. The language often seems dead and unimaginative. Words or phrases seem to be assumed as at one with a singular meaning, complete and self-explanatory. There is often little discussion of the assumptions made in the research questions and the methods. Most importantly, the figure is lifted from its ground, meaning context is completely lost. The problem is that research is now the absolute dominant language in which art therapy is being developed. Like capitalism, there seems to be no alternative.

DISCUSSION

Fisher (2009) asserts that in order to have any political agency we have to accept our 'insertion at the level of desire in the remorseless meat-grinder of capital' (p. 15). On the one hand capitalism is an abstract system we feel powerless within, but on the other hand, it wouldn't exist if we were not complicit in it. Later, he says:

> however much individuals or groups may have disdained or ironised the language of competition, entrepreneurialism and consumerism that has been installed in UK institutions since the 1980s, our widespread ritualistic compliance with this terminology has served to naturalise the dominance of capital and helped to neutralise any opposition to it.
>
> (Fisher, 2011, p. 124)

By highlighting art therapy's limits and acknowledging therapists' self-interest, we are not arguing against art therapy. Rather, we argue that art therapists find a way to work within the system that does not collude with its values. We think, like Fisher (2011), that this can be done by showing up where the incontrovertible logic of neoliberalism is untenable. Fisher gives examples: how can the free market improve our lives when profiteering leads to climate catastrophe? Capitalism cannot survive without workers, yet there is a refusal to acknowledge this dependence; robots may be cheaper, but without people what is the work for?

Contradictions are not in themselves the problem. In fact, contradiction is at the heart of creativity in the form of dialectics. Whilst Hegel had recognised humans' propensity to develop through the reconciling or synthesising of contradictions, the synthesis then producing further contradictions, and that human enlightenment was the goal, Marx saw the material coming first in the dialectic. Thus, the dialectic is formed in relation to our transforming the matter of the world into things useful to us, like food. The dialectic is in the opposing struggle between the owners of the means of production, who can reap the profit from the workers' labour because of that ownership, whilst the workers get only what they are given, their power being resistance. Psychoanalysts recognised dialectical processes in the binaries of conscious/unconscious, the depressive and paranoid positions, the individual and community. Post-structuralists and phenomenologists such as Merleau-Ponty, who prioritised the body in relation to contradictions, and Derrida, who unpicked texts to show up their contradictions, all saw contradiction as the basis of creativity, the urge to reconcile opposites which can never be fully resolved but that bring about development through creating further oppositions.

The feminist bell hooks, writing in 1982, speaks of the contradiction that feminists have structured a women's liberation movement that is racist and excludes many non-white women. She quotes from an anonymous women's liberation pamphlet:

> In all these struggles we must be assertive and challenging, combatting the deep seated tendency in Americans to be liberal, that is, to evade struggling over questions of principle for fear of creating tensions or becoming unpopular. Instead we must live by the fundamental dialectical principle: that progress comes only from struggling to resolve contradictions.
>
> (p. 195)

The next chapter looks at how art therapists have engaged in the political struggle in their art therapy group practice.

REFERENCES

BAAT (2021). *About Art Therapy* [online]. Available at: https://www.baat.org/About-Art-Therapy [Accessed 14th July 2021].

Bateman, A. and Fonagy, P. (2013). Mentalization-based treatment. *Psychoanalytic inquiry*, 33(6), pp. 595–613.

Dalal, F. (2016). Group analysis in the time of austerity: Neo-liberalism, managerialism and evidence-based research. *Group Analysis*, 50(1), pp. 35–54.

Dalal, F. (2018). *CBT: The Cognitive Behavioural Tsunami: Managerialism, Politics and the Corruptions of Science*. 1st ed., London and New York: Routledge.

de Boettie, E. (1577). *Discours de la servitude volontaire*, Editions Mille et une nuits, 1997. ISBN 2-910233-94-4.

Fisher, M. (2009). *Capitalist Realism: Is There No Alternative?* Hampshire: John Hunt Publishing.

Fisher, M. (2011). The privatisation of stress. *Soundings*, 48, pp. 123–133.

Fisher, M. (2012). 'Why mental health is a political issue'. *The Guardian*, 16th July [online]. Available at: https://www.theguardian.com/commentisfree/2012/jul/16/mental-health-political-issue [Accessed 29th June 2021].

Foulkes, S.H. and Anthony, E.J. (1965). *Group Psychotherapy: The Psychoanalytic Approach*. 2nd ed., London and New York: Routledge.

Franks, M. and Whitaker, R. (2007). The image, mentalisation and group art psychotherapy. *International Journal of Art Therapy: Inscape*, 12(1), pp. 3–16.

Fuller, P.R. (2013). *Surviving, Existing, or Living: Phase-Specific Therapy for Severe Psychosis*. London and New York: Routledge.

Gill, B. (2019). *The Great NHS Heist* [video]. Available at: https://www.youtube.com/watch?v=kwlvLe-X27o [Accessed 29th June 2021].

Gilroy, A. (2006). *Art therapy, Research and Evidence-Based Practice*. London, California and New Delhi: Sage.

Gipson, L. (2017). Challenging neoliberalism and multicultural love in art therapy. *Art Therapy*, 34(3), pp. 112–117.

Hakim, J., Chatzidakis, A., Littler, J., Rottenberg, C. and Segal, L. (2020). *The Care Manifesto*. 1st ed., London: Verso.

Havsteen-Franklin, D. and Altamirano, J.C. (2015). Containing the uncontainable: Responsive art making in art therapy as a method to facilitate mentalization. *International Journal of Art Therapy*, 20(2), pp. 54–65.

HCPC (2014). *Standards of education*. HCPC [online]. Available at: https://www.hcpc-uk.org/resources/standards/standards-of-education-and-training/ [Accessed 29th June 2021].

hooks, b. (1982). *Ain't I a Woman, Black Women and Feminism*. London: Pluto Press.

Huet, V. (2012). Creativity in a cold climate: Art therapy-based organisational consultancy within public healthcare. *International Journal of Art Therapy*, 17(1), pp. 25–33.

Huet, V. and Holttum, S. (2016). Art therapy-based groups for work-related stress with staff in health and social care: An exploratory study. *The Arts in Psychotherapy*, 50, pp. 46–57.

Marshall-Tierney, A. (2014). Making art with and without patients in acute settings. *International Journal of Art Therapy*, 19(3), pp. 96–106.

Millar, S.L., Chambers, M. and Giles, M. (2016). Service user involvement in mental health care: An evolutionary concept analysis. *Health Expectations*, 19(2), pp. 209–221.

Morgan, L., Knight, C., Bagwash, J. and Thompson, F. (2012). Borderline personality disorder and the role of art therapy: A discussion of its utility from the perspective of those with a lived experience. *International Journal of Art Therapy*, 17(3), pp. 91–97.

Or, M.B. (2010). Clay sculpting of mother and child figures encourages mentalization. *The Arts in Psychotherapy*, 37(4), pp. 319–327.

Rothwell, K. and Grandison, S. (2016). Notes on Service Design for Art Psychotherapists Working in Time-Limited Group Programmes on Adult Mental Health Inpatient Wards. In: Hughes, R. (ed.), *Time-Limited Art Psychotherapy: Developments in Theory and Practice*, 1st ed., Oxon and New York: Routledge, pp.180–194.

Smail, D.J. (2005). *Power, Interest and Psychology: Elements of a Social Materialist Understanding of Distress*. Monmouth: PCCS Books.

Springham, N. and Camic, P.M. (2017). Observing mentalizing art therapy groups for people diagnosed with borderline personality disorder. *International Journal of Art Therapy*, 22(3), pp. 138–152.

Springham, N. and Huet, V. (2020). Facing our shadows: Understanding harm in the arts therapies. *International Journal of Art Therapy*, 25(1), pp. 5–18.

Springham, N., Findlay, D., Woods, A. and Harris, J. (2012). How can art therapy contribute to mentalization in borderline personality disorder? *International Journal of Art Therapy*, 17(3), pp. 115–129.

Tipple, R. (2017). Thinking versus mentalization. *Art Therapy OnLine*, 8(2).

Walton, F. (2016). Art Therapy in the NHS and in Private Practice. In: West, J. (ed.), *Art Therapy in Private Practice: Theory, Practice and Research in Changing Contexts*. 1st ed., London and Philadelphia: Jessica Kingsley Publishers, pp. 56–75.

Wood, C. (2013). In the wake of the Matisse RCT: What about art therapy and psychosis? *International Journal of Art Therapy*, 18(3), pp. 88–97.

Wood, C. (2020). Hearing Voices Movement and art therapy. *Art Therapy*, 37(2), pp. 88–92.

Woods, A. and Springham, N. (2012). On learning from being the in-patient. *International Journal of Art Therapy*, 16(2), pp. 60–68.

CHAPTER THREE

Art therapy as resistance

Sally Skaife and Jon Martyn

DOI: 10.4324/9781003107408-4

INTRODUCTION

The changes imposed on institutions by neoliberalism do not work in the interests of those that implement them and certainly do not work for those affected by them. However, despite this, art therapists can end up ignoring the contradictions that neoliberalism produces and colluding with its ideological trends, such as the individualising of suffering and the promotion of hyper-rationality. In the last chapter we argued that it was important that we stay alert to the contradictions, as this will engage us in a struggle to resolve them, which is a political or class struggle. When we speak of class, we are speaking of a dynamic between those that benefit from neoliberalism and those that do not. This includes consideration of intersecting modes of domination, such as race and gender, in which some benefit from others' disadvantage (Olufemi, 2020).

The psychoanalyst Lynne Layton (2019) explores the conflicted position white people have in relation to race. She talks of whites of privilege wanting to hide from the pain of acknowledging that our advantages have been, and continue to be, at the expense of those who have been exploited by colonialism and slavery and its continuation in intersectional inequality. Simultaneously, we also have a desire to face this pain so that we can integrate what has become split off but which still continues to haunt us. Art therapists may come from different places from one another in relation to 'class', but we share one aspect of the dynamic, the danger of splitting off what feels too difficult, projecting it into our clients and then dealing with it in our therapeutic work with 'the other'. In doing this we end up performing in the interests of neoliberalism.

In this chapter we consider the way in which class relations manifest in the ambiguous and contradictory relations involved in art and therapy. We start with a discussion of the ways in which art therapy has tended historically to deal with contradiction, that is, by polarisation. An example being the names; art psychotherapy often referring to groups in which there is verbal reflection, and art therapy referring to those that privilege art making. We argue that, if instead contradictions are exposed, a struggle to reconcile them can engage the group in a political process.

This thinking is related to some selected group art therapy papers that are examples of literature that acknowledge art therapy as taking place within systems of class conflict. Looking at these selected pieces in their context within various art therapy traditions gives a deeper understanding of how art therapists are working with the contradictions of neoliberalism.

We have broadened our lens in this chapter to look beyond the UK and also outside mainstream institutions. In the UK, art therapy is widening its field in response to cutbacks in mainstream services. It now crosses into territories it once made efforts to be distinct from, moving into wellbeing, general health, arts in health, community and social projects, as well as educational frames. Mental health services have been delivered in museums and galleries (Schaer et al., 2008, Coles and Jury, 2020) and the natural environment (Heginworth and Nash, 2019). In the US and Canada, Expressive Arts, which works with all art forms and with a primarily social focus, has always had a broader reach; it now seems Social Action and Social Justice art therapy are in a similar field, with attention put in at a 'macro' (social) level to boost the health of communities in order to help individuals within them (Kapitan et al., 2011). There appear to be many more similarities between art therapy in the UK and US now in comparison to the past, and there is a growing art therapy literature from outside the UK and US. However, early differences have continued to characterise approaches between either side of the Atlantic and are thus prevalent in art therapy literature as a whole, which cannot help but have been influenced by them.

SPLITS IN ART THERAPY

Observations at American Art Therapy Association (AATA) conferences (Gilroy and Skaife, 1997) revealed that the US and the UK had widely different art therapy practices, but in both cases there were clear splits. In the US, art was, on the one hand, an adjunct to psychology used diagnostically and tied to specific art-based interventions. On the other, art was seen as linked to spiritual healing, with the art therapist as a powerful, charismatic person, a sort of shaman. It appeared that therapeutic work in both types of art therapy was almost entirely oriented towards changing feelings viewed as negative (anger, sadness) into positive feelings – rage and depression seemed out of the question. This contrasted to the UK idea of art therapy that it was a space in which difficult feelings could reach expression and be worked with.

In the UK, there was a split between psychoanalytically based group models and the art as healing mode. The former saw therapist(s), patient(s) and art in a dynamic relationship in which roles could be explored, but often the process of art making went unrecognised in favour of the appreciation of symbols and representations. In the latter, art was seen as transformational, but the relationships which determined the art and the way in which it is looked at went unremarked. As studios closed down another split emerged between psychodynamic practice and that based on human theory, the latter often addressing social issues more overtly, but as in the art as healing mode, the therapist was assumed as an unexplored benign presence and the work kept in the conscious realm, often with directives.

Thus, in both countries we could describe art therapy as 'ethnocentric monoculturalism' (Talwar, 2018). Whilst class conflict seemed disallowed in US art therapy, in the UK there was a tendency for art therapy to ignore social and political realities in favour of power relations reduced to transference and countertransference, and 'here and now' interpersonal relationships (Brooks, 1999), or, in the models based on human theory, to disregard the way in which power relations played out within the therapy itself. It seemed that the US psychology-based model was related to the limits of licensure (art therapy not being recognised as a profession) and requirements of a health system paid for through insurance, in which packages of treatments were connected to particular diagnoses. As we saw in the last chapter, the gradual privatisation of public services in the UK has led art therapy to become more linked to diagnoses and manualised treatments here too.

By the end of the 1990s, literature in both the US (Junge et al.,1993, McNiff, 1997, Moon, 1997, and Kaplan, 2000) and UK (Schaverien, 1994, Dalley, 2000, Maclagan, 2001) spoke of polarities around approaches to the combining of 'art' and 'therapy', and proposed dynamic balance and integration. Maxine Junge, Janise Finn Alvarez, Anne Kellogg and Christine Volker (1993), though, had a political take, seeing the art therapist in a double bind, embodying both the psychotherapist, who they saw as a stalwart of the status quo who attempts to confine and exclude those who don't conform, and the artist, who makes waves and helps society to see and feel injustice and imagine something better. Junge et al.'s view has echoes of Waller's (2004) idea of art therapists as pragmatic rebels.

During the following two decades polarities gave way to plurality. Both Susan Hogan (2009), UK, and Ephrat Huss (2009), Israel, give an overview of different art therapy models, Hogan describing six types ranging from using art as a tool in a psychotherapeutic relationship, to art making with only minimal verbal intervention. Huss describes a prism, the sides seeming to refer to different lenses rather than different models as all describe a similar mode which involves interventions, therapist skills and art therapy techniques, and thus is a rejection of more psychodynamic modes of working. Hogan's later publication (2015) describes a wide range of approaches reflecting pluralism or a fragmentation of art therapy, depending on how you look at it. Only three of the nine models give consideration to the embodied political: group-interactive, feminist and social art therapy.

These are descriptive observations of the different art therapy practices prevalent at the time of their writing. There is a danger though that if we embrace an idea of different models applicable to different clients and contexts, we avoid the tensions that exist in all art therapy groups between different class viewpoints. The reproduction of class relations is inevitable in any group; not addressing them is an option, but as these processes are present in the group, this denial is, in itself, a very active, powerful intervention.

WORKING WITH CONTRADICTION IN ART THERAPY

In attempting in my own art therapy practice (Sally) to avoid colluding and replicating dominating practices, I have been drawn to thinking of the deconstruction of binaries. Art therapy can replicate hierarchical splits from constructed mind/body divisions. The cognitive, logic and thinking have been split off and valued over the perceptual, aesthetic and feeling, as if, for example, thinking did not involve feeling and logic was not aesthetic, and exploited for political reasons, as we have seen with audit and evaluation. Mind/body splits in art therapy between the cognitive and the perceptual parallel those that have become associated with hierarchies of people. For example, the upper and middle classes are thought to use their minds, whilst the working class use their bodies in labour, women catering for the bodily needs of the labourers and producing the next generation of workers; in racism, skin colour and facial features are used to divide and subjugate, and in gender, the female body is objectified and abused. These power relations permeate our unconscious and so emerge in our groups. Binary making, in itself though, is ubiquitous, and as Derrida (1988) argues, binaries are always hierarchical. Binaries in art therapy can mirror one another; art/talk, play/work, black/white, therapist/client. These can represent opposing forces at any one time; that is, the voice that speaks dominant ideology and the voice that is repressed or opposes it. Deconstruction picks up what does not fit into either category, thus disrupting the binary. These voices were represented in my own practice in the different experiences of black and white people.

In a supervision group that I ran on an art therapy training course (Skaife, 2007), two different positions, experienced between black students and white students in response to a clinical dilemma about the racial make-up of a children's group, were represented by silence on the one hand, and talking on the other. The obvious thing seemed to be to interpret the black student's silence as anger, but this did not seem right. Instead, I did nothing, allowing an irresolvable conundrum, a new contradiction with the group's purpose of discussing clinical work. Later, when I reflected on it, I thought of the silence as being like a blank painting, that spoke of absence through its presence. The absence I thought of as the absence of a resolution to the legacy of colonialism. I understood this dynamic to relate to Pat Parker's aphorism, 'The first thing you do is to forget that I'm Black. Second, you must never forget that I'm Black' (1978). In a later paper (Skaife, 2013), I deconstructed my process notes from a group I ran with asylum seekers, in which I was white and the group members were black. I found that exploring the way in which one side of any binary is inherent in the other (white only exists in relation to black and vice versa) enabled a continuous shifting of lens between a dominant position and a subjugated one, the aim being to give prominence to what becomes hidden whilst showing up the inter-reliance of the two positions. The art therapist Sheridan Linnell (2010) also deconstructs gender and race and the therapist/client relationship in art therapy in the postcolonial context of Australia.

With these ideas in mind, we turn to examine some art therapy literature. The issue is in what ways do art therapists, who have an overt interest in working with social and political issues, handle contradictions that may emerge in art, dialogue or in the therapeutic relationship in their art therapy groups? We have selected papers that address community interventions, as it is in this work that there has been an active attempt to avoid the individualising and pathologising of mental distress. Community interventions enable greater recognition of our position within political systems of domination and present the opportunity of facing outwards, recognising the personal in the political and vice versa. The following papers were chosen as representing different approaches to this. We include papers we have been involved in writing to place the developing themes of this book in context in the literature.

We have divided the papers into three categories. The first is where the therapist leaves a Western country to work with a population that has been exploited by Western imperialism, and thus, herself,[1] clearly

---

1 We use the feminine to refer to all genders in this section of text.

embodies a power relation with those with whom she will work. The second category is those art therapists that are working on their own turf and may come from the same community as those they work with. The papers here describe work where the therapy has moved outside the usual therapeutic space. The last category is where the therapist is working in an institution and therefore the therapy is likely to be replicating the power relations of that institution.

FROM THE COUNTRIES OF COLONISERS TO THOSE THAT HAVE BEEN COLONISED

Art therapists who travel from the Western world to populations in other countries exploited by Western imperialism unavoidably carry the power of the oppressor, in their internalised world as well as in what they will represent to those with whom they will work. This is also true of the art therapy intervention that they bring.

Lynn Kapitan, Mary Litell and Anabell Torres (2011) describe a cross-cultural collaboration in a long-term participatory arts-based research project in Nicaragua. The project was created both by, and for, grassroots community organisers in Nicaragua and funded through a non-governmental organisation (NGO). The authors are keenly aware of the way in which the Western world has dominated and exploited countries like Nicaragua, creating wars and poverty. They attempt to ensure that they are not exporting ethnocentric art therapy techniques through drawing on local culture and aesthetics, and are interested in what Latin American culture can offer to decolonise western perspectives. The project draws on Paulo Friere's educational model, which favours learning that comes from within the community themselves. 'Conscientizacao' (consciousness raising) underpinned structured group art making, with symbolic and archetypal associations to images enabling dialogue around social issues. A collective image is made of some evocative cultural symbols, and a volcano with a hat becomes a central representation of a community's response to both their living by a volcano and to its symbolism for their experiences of repression, eruption, adaptation and transformation of emotional life. A task to explore the dynamics of the roles of creator, destroyer and transformer, with participants taking it in turns to create and destroy and remake each other's artworks, was introduced. The intention was that these structured activities could be replicated with the participants' communities, which might then strengthen a community's capacity to take political action.

The paper describes a structured intervention associated with a conceptual frame. The next example is a contrast in that art making appears more spontaneous and unpredictable in nature.

Carrie MacLeod's paper (2011), coming from an Expressive Arts tradition, is based on the idea that art in itself can transform conflict. Here the cognitive/perceptive hierarchical binary is upended, with the perceptual, aesthetic and imaginative given prominence. MacLeod, a Canadian art therapist, describes a project in a remote community in Sierra Leone, a decade after the civil war, in which the community's youth were engaged in creating ideas for a collaborative arts project. Fed up with the negative picture of Sierra Leone, a country which struggles with poverty and the dreadful after-effects of war, the young people were keen to do something celebratory and decided on creating a Peace Festival. This was to be an inter-ethnic festival that combined three modes: cultural art forms, traditional practices and expressive arts. MacLeod describes the different sorts of contributions made, such as a boy with amputated legs developing a 'choreography of absence', a dance performance standing on his hands that expresses both 'elation and mourning' (p. 154). The rehearsals sound rich but difficult, with themes including, losses, fears and anger of war, which MacLeod writes about as emanating from the art forms themselves. Amongst the otherwise willing participants was a group of self-proclaimed 'outsiders', hostile to foreign peace interventions, including arts-based ones, who were tired of government initiatives that promoted peace and reconciliation. They explained that 'forced forgiveness and reconciliation is an abhorrent crime' … 'lingering hostilities cannot be casually bypassed' and … 'idealism is nothing but another form of violence in disguise' (MacLeod, 2011, p. 150). MacLeod gave scope for the outsider group to subvert the festival's message, and they used puppets to amplify and mock their fellow villagers and ironically acted out governmental 'truth and reconciliation' protocols, to which the community/audience responded with infectious laughter.

Although MacLeod (2011) does not refer within this paper to coming from a privileged country, or of her whiteness in relation to the black young people, the 'outsider' group were making references to it when speaking of unhelpful foreigners' peace initiatives. MacLeod's work, as expressive arts, is ambiguously related to therapy; the book that it is in refers to art therapy in its title, but MacLeod does not refer to her work as therapy. However, it is clear she regards it as having a powerful therapeutic effect on its participants, as well as providing the social forum for oppressions to become communally felt.

Our last example of this section (Lloyd and Usiskin, 2020) describes a project in which two art therapists from Art Refuge, an NGO/charity, travel from the UK to work with migrants in the French–UK border town of Calais. It is an environment where migrants are subject to regular police violence, often having all their belongings removed, including shoes and personal items, as well as to gangs running trafficking and sexual exploitation operations.

Art Refuge, working in partnership with humanitarian organisations such as Medicines San Frontiers, Médecins du Monde and Secours Catholique, has had a presence in Calais since 2015; at the time of this paper, going there for 2 days a fortnight. The work engages participants of mainly Middle Eastern and North African descent who are attempting to cross the English Channel to claim asylum in the UK. Bobby Lloyd and Miriam Usiskin (2020) describe the construction of a map, co-created with migrants. Unable to use their usual space, the therapists move the map outside, creating a three-dimensional space by moving the location of the map to different places into which people come and go, having conversations in response to the map about journeys, disorientation and having nowhere to belong. On the way home the therapists frequently ask themselves what they are doing there, and their reflections end up as a blog posted on social media along with images. These are shared with, and contributed to, by the migrants and supporters, as well as other refugees visiting the social media sites. The blogs aim is to give the marginalised some control over how they are represented, to educate and to challenge demeaning stereotypes. Above all, the work emphasises that art making can 'encourage leaps of imagination and hope for something better' (p. 140).

Lloyd and Usiskin (2020) say, 'Often at the map, we ourselves feel deskilled, demoralised and carrying a profound sense of shame, which is in part our own countertransference both to those we work with and the context' (p. 136). This shame seems linked to the profound difference that they can get on a train and return to the UK with ease, whereas the migrants have to risk their lives to attempt it. This sounds extremely difficult and a moment when they were able to face the pain of the dynamic relation of their privilege.

All three papers show that the colonial/race power dynamic is present in the work though related to differently. In Kapitan et al.'s work (2011) much preparation has gone into ensuring that dominating practices are avoided. In MacLeod's paper (2011) the relationship is represented through the art, though MacLeod does not discuss this as a reference to her therapist role and identity, which leaves questions as to whether or not the work should be thought of as therapy. Lloyd and Usiskin (2020) refer to a conscious working through of the power dynamic in their social media processing. All these projects appear to have been short term, over a few days. In the following section, longer term projects are possible.

IN THE LOCALITY

In this section we describe art therapy work where the therapist is not travelling to work with the global poor but working either within their own community or in the same city. This enables a sharing between therapist and clients of experiences of marginalisation. As with the papers in the previous section there is a community focus and the projects involve leaving the art therapy studio. This opens up questions relating to boundaries.

Salamishah Tillet and Scheherezade Tillet (2018) describe a year-long artist activist programme set up to empower African-American teen girls in Chicago to advocate for gender and racial equality, and against violence towards women and girls, in their communities and beyond. The project was called 'A Long Walk Home', and was a Chicago-based national non-profit. Many of these girls were traumatised having experienced police, community, domestic and sexual violence, or been witness to it in their area of Chicago. The art therapists, who were also African-American, chose a black feminist rubric self-care as a model of art therapy. To enter into the programme each girl produced an art portfolio that reflected the various forms of art expressions present in their homes and communities: hair braiding, rapping and stepping, creative writing, photography, dance and visual art. Classes on gender and equality invited the students to share their stories, and students were given an individual therapist where appropriate. The girls were given journals and cameras so that they could document their lives through monologues and self-portraits. This stage was called Girl/Me. They moved on to Girl/Culture, in which they thought about how their experiences were shared by others. An exhibition entitled, 'The Visibility Project: A Celebration of 100 Black Girls', which featured the artwork they had made on the project, was held at the School of the Art Institute of Chicago. Lastly, in Girl/Power, they upended the marketised, individualised and thus antifeminist and racist concept of 'self-care' by considering self-care as involving it interdependence and political resistance. At a Domestic Violence Awareness march, which commemorated the life of an unarmed young woman shot in the back of the head by a police officer, they handed out leaflets they had made that included self-portraits of themselves, thus joining themselves to a larger collective and dissolving the boundaries of politicised violence and personalised trauma.

There are echoes of the Kapitan et al. (2011) approach in the cognitively devised directives of this work. The shared identity of therapists and clients (black, female) enabled powerful work, but the use of directives, as well as the difference in ages and social capital, must have meant that there was a power dynamic within the therapy that appears to not have been explored. If it had though, the powerful feelings that could have emerged might have made leaving the therapy space feel unsafe. The next project appears to leave space for class dynamics to emerge.

Hayley Berman (2017) describes the development of Lefika, an NGO in South Africa founded in black neighbourhoods marginalised and traumatised by apartheid. As well as providing art therapy, Lefika trains local community workers in art counselling based on group psychoanalytic thinking. The aim is that in helping the community workers to process experiences of trauma, they become able to take on parental roles for orphaned and neglected children that are sorely needed. Berman describes two group art therapy spaces set up in response to rising anti-migrant violence that led to people needing placement in refugee camps. Being aware of how past trauma, here of experiences in apartheid, gets repressed and repeated in violence towards 'the other', the therapists' aim is for spaces where the repressed can be shared and held socially. They use a mix of social dreaming (the communal sharing of dreams without comment or analysis) and art making for processing their experiences. Into the dreams come images of the horrendous violence from the apartheid past as well as the xenophobic present, mixed with references to current poverty and neglect. The participants follow up the dreams with art making, which brings together the dream images with universal images of childhood and nourishment, for example, which can be reflected on.

This paper illustrates a way of working in which art making, social dreaming and reflection are brought together to enable the processing of painful repressed material. 'The hosts' see themselves as holding the fragments together, processing the feelings engendered in them by the material in separate spaces, and a movement back and forth between returning to the rawness of the material and to reflective thinking about it. The last example in this set also involves work with refugees, but in the UK.

'Najma', Tania Kaczynski, Jon Martyn and Emma Hollamby (2021) describe a one-day-a-week group art therapy space for asylum seekers, New Art Studio, in which therapists and members make art together. The focus is on reconnection with imagination and what has become repressed, on being with others, inhabiting an alternative identity to the pejorative 'asylum seeker', and asserting one's existence through the making of marks. The studio puts on exhibitions as part of the therapy, all being involved (if they wish) in the framing, curation, promotion and selling of the work. After an exhibition, group members return to the studio space to discuss and process the experience. 'Najma' et al. describe several important dynamics that are brought to the fore by the exhibiting: the artwork can speak for itself, thereby protecting the artist; it can educate the public about the plight of asylum seekers; it can redress the demeaning stereotypes about them; it can bring self-esteem to the artists; and it can give them a different identify than one with a lack. The authors describe the experience of the exhibition as raising feelings of competition, failure and inequality for members, but they are encouraged to express and explore these.

Whether or not art therapists work in a colonised country or share a similar identity to their clients, the clients are always 'other' in some way by virtue of the role. Each of these papers have considered this differently. Tillet and Tillet (2018) don't mention it. Berman (2017), though she explores inequality, doesn't mention her own position, a white therapist working with black clients, a mirror of the relations in post-apartheid South Africa that are the focus of the paper. 'Najma' et al. (2021), like Kapitan et al. (2011), attempt to even out the power within the structure of the therapy. Interestingly, their making the client first author of the paper speaks to this power relation. Contradiction is apparent in the 'Najma' et al. paper in relation to the exhibition, which presents the studio members as artists, whilst interest in the exhibition may be to do with the art being that of asylum seekers. There is a reflection of the 'First forget I'm black, second never forget I'm black' saying which captures the dynamic to which all the papers have a position. Remember we are equal, but don't forget that we exist within a system of oppression in which you are privileged at my expense.

IN MAINSTREAM INSTITUTIONS

As we saw in the previous chapters, neoliberal ideology pervades our institutions. As art therapy takes place within this system, without active subversion it inevitably replicates it. This was very much on the minds of the art therapists in this section.

In a London NHS trust, Jane Dudley (2011) describes an art therapy median group of up to twenty mental health users, which was open to whoever wished to attend, regardless of their level of distress or diagnosis. Participants made work as they chose. Dudley considers the median group as a community, as inpatients and outpatients who attended had often met before through repeated admissions; this helped lessen the sense of us and them, as all belonged to the community of the service, including all the staff. She emphasised to group members that the group worked because of what each individually brought to it. She thought of the group as a microcosm of society, 'by thinking large we can hold the larger group in mind' (p. 4). Dudley felt that an emphasis on the group as a whole, and on group members taking responsibility for passing the culture on to newer members, was a central factor in the group's eventual high and stable attendance. She speaks of resisting the temptation to always find words to talk about the art, as expression without words within a responsive community can be a relief from the pressure to talk that can be experienced in other parts of the hospital. Dudley discusses her reasons for not making art herself in the group and remaining seated during the art making. She was consciously allowing the power relation to be present in the group, but without it being a dominating one. The group had extremely positive feedback from its members but despite its success was closed down. Group members decided to protest at its closure, which Dudley says indicated that the aim had been achieved.

This same group model that Dudley uses informs the Art Therapy Large Group run on the MA Art Psychotherapy programme at Goldsmiths, University of London. The large group is seen as a community space, enabling a shared encounter to which the whole learning community is able to relate. Art making, performance and dialogue in the group enables representation and the processing of social and political issues, as well as issues relating to equality and diversity, and professional development. The group, to which all the staff and students attend (around 100 people), has no explicit agenda, and often invokes powerful feelings of hate and fear; the idea is that these can be transformed through the group process, modelling the challenge of transforming society from a hierarchically driven one to a democratic one.

Sally Skaife, Lesley Morris, Robin Tipple and Diana Velada's (2020) paper follows the story of a camera that the staff introduced for the group's use for the purposes of a research project. The paper describes a conflict in which students were ambivalent about the research and the camera. Responses to the camera, in the form of different material representations, dialogue and performance, seemed to be ways in which participants brought the staff–student power relation to the surface of the group material, where it echoed other class relations that emerged in the group. The repeated iterations in relation to the camera are understood by the authors to be ways in which the group made the cathected object their own in a form of resistance. The authors describe the group space as similar to a theatre or a heterotopia, a space outside of real time in which incompatible spaces are brought together in a real space (Foucault, 2000). In this group there were political demonstrations, family sitting rooms and an area affected by a tsunami.

Although the students were invited to contribute to the research on the group, they were not co-participants; the research team were concerned about a conflict with their roles as assessors. However, they also thought their not abdicating the role of power enabled visibility of relations of power in education. There were clear contradictions here in relation to their espoused aim for the group, that is, of lateral relating, when the students were not able to achieve equality in relation to the research and therefore could only expose the power relation or subvert it.

Dudley's group ran counter to the institution's values and was closed down. Skaife et al.'s paper grapples with the dilemma of needing evidence of the effectiveness of the mode of education to satisfy institutional demands, which then runs counter to the idea of the group's purpose.

DISCUSSION

We have been arguing that art therapy has the potential to subvert neoliberalism through attending to its contradictions, and with these papers we have been looking at whether or not contradictions in the therapist's power in relation to the clients is ignored, smoothed over or openly addressed. It appears that the differences between the papers can be related to the art therapy traditions from which they come. Both Kapitan et al.,'s (2011) and Tillet and Tillet's (2018) papers come from a Social Action, Social Justice tradition in the US, in which the intention is to create new ways of working. Talwar (2018) speaks of consciously planned acts of resistance which disrupt the established order, for example, naming people differently or talking back; and through reclaiming public spaces, reclaiming agency and the ability to assert empowered identities. It is perhaps in line with this that both Kapitan et al. and Tillet and Tillet use structured approaches, ensuring an art making practice that is not at odds with their conceptual aims for the group. Kapitan et al. consciously attempt to ensure an equality of power in the work. Tillet and Tillet have a shared identity with their clients. In making their clients' voices heard, they make their own voices heard, redressing the system of domination that has silenced them.

There is a contradiction in Kapitan et al.,'s paper. The exercise in which, in groups of three, one made an artwork, another destroyed it and a third repaired it split off the suffering that defined the exercise. That is, the pain of having something you've made destroyed (mirroring destruction from violence or the eruption of a volcano) was not experienced because you knew in advance that what you made would be torn up. In its place was 'glee', enjoyment at the play involved. Further in the paper they talk of a crayon replacing a machete. This binary is used to embody the notion of suffering and violence, as represented by the machete, being replaced with the empowering and fulfilling nature of art, as represented by the crayon. There is violence, though, involved in the process of art making; we ourselves might destroy what we make, or feel despair at our production, but then find a way to repair it, or not.

MacLeod's (2011) Sierra Leone Peace Project is in the Expressive Arts tradition. Originating in Canada and the US, Expressive Arts practitioners, who use all the art forms, consider that artistic expression, in itself, is transformational (Levine, 1992). They think that it is the world rather than the individual that needs changing but believe this can come about through the healing power of art, both for individuals and the collective (Estrella, 2011). This approach certainly redresses the privilege given to cognition in approaches to mental suffering, but does it fall into a mind/body split and so disguise the power relation? If the 'outsider group' had not been there in MacLeod's work, maybe the group's reaction to MacLeod's identity, as a white professional from the West, a representative of the imperialism responsible for the suffering of the marginalised poor black youth she was working with, would not have emerged at all.

Lloyd and Usiskin (2020), Berman (2017), 'Najma' et al. (2021), Dudley (2011) and Skaife et al. (2020) define their projects in relation to a psychodynamic approach, which instead of structured art making according to cognitive ideas, allows the process to go as it will, which inevitably will result in power difference becoming present in the therapy, though it may not be commented on. Dudley and Skaife et al.'s papers present the therapist as consciously performing roles of authority, with the idea coming from the psychoanalytic tradition that these can be deconstructed or analysed. Lloyd and Usiskin describe their work as drawing on Social Action as well as psychoanalytic traditions.

Contradictions emerge too in the research that some of the papers address. Though participatory action-based research, as used by Kapitan et al. (2011), Berman (2017) and Lloyd and Usiskin (2020), does offer a good model for avoiding exploitation and allows art forms as data, there is a question as to how far any research starts to limit the practice, requiring a sort of tidying up of material. We, Skaife et al. (2020), using different research methods, found ourselves caught in a paradox in which the objective method was at odds with the subjective experience of what was being researched. The turn to a subjectively based model, based on observational drawing, raises the question as to whether or not the project could or should be considered research, as replicability could never produce the same 'findings'. Lloyd and Usiskin (2020) talk of more research needed on art materials, which seems to suggest there is an aim for 'best practice'. Berman says:

> The Lefika model of practice is highly replicable, portable, cost effective and relevant in helping to address the multitude of trauma we are confronting on a global level as a social enterprise.
>
> (2017, p. 6)

In suggesting the projects are replicable, there is a denial of their particularity in a context, in which even those not directly involved in it are in fact contributing to it. There is a contradiction. If the intention is that community art therapy work is about inclusivity and empowerment of those involved, then each project needs to be co-created from its inception.

As we have said, contradictions are always present whether we expose them or not.

It may be that suppression of the 'here and now', that is, open discussion of feelings in relation to others in the present, is felt necessary for doing the work in some cases. In the foreword to Levine and Levine's (2011) book, '*Art in Action: Expressive Art Therapy and Social Change*', in which MacLeod's paper is a chapter, Michelle LeBaron writes, 'Focusing on the issues in conflict often escalates disagreement, worsens relationships and deepens the conflict itself' (p. 11). If we push away conflict though, are we avoiding the pain of class exploitation, leaving it to be silently experienced by the marginalised?

The politically orientated papers we have discussed have illustrated differences between the US and UK art therapy traditions. In the US there is an attempt to avoid the repetition of domination that is associated with art therapy methods, which rely on pathologising individuals, by doing art therapy differently. The UK papers draw more on those aspects of the psychoanalytic tradition, which allow for conflict to be alive in the group. A difference in the histories of the countries might give one explanation for this. In the US, violence has been at home in the form of the slaughter of the indigenous population and in slavery. Nowadays, gun violence is a tangible part of daily life for many Americans. In the UK, where the violence of colonialism has been meted out on foreign soils, its history frequently denied. Where violence is in contemporary life, it is a marginalised experience, ignored or unknown to a majority. Conflict in the UK may be more alive in the group, but often this is understood only in relation to family or in-group relationships rather than as the legacy of its history of colonialism and the violence of continued class oppression.

Not only are there differences between each side of the Atlantic though, there are differences within them. In North America we have the directive approach of Kapitan et al. and Tillet and Tillet, and the Expressive Arts approach of MacLeod. Within the UK, too, there are differences still between more directive art therapy groups, which often address overtly political themes related to gender or other forms of oppression, for example, Liebmann (1994, 1997,) Liebmann and Ward (1999), Hogan (1997, 2018), Jones et al. (1999), and those which are more group analytically based, for example, Canty (2009), Melliar and Bruhka (2010) and Dudley (2011).

Other differences were apparent in the length of group interventions, whether or not group members left the art therapy space and the difference between community-based interventions and small groups. Additionally, the different positions of therapists of colour and white therapists implies different viewpoints, the former, though, getting written out of dominant art therapy discourses (Talwar, 2018, Gipson, 2018).

CONCLUSION

Both Layton (2019) and Parker (1978) speak of a contradiction, that is oppositional forces. Layton is talking of this contradiction in relation to white people wanting and not wanting to face the fact that their privilege is at the expense of black people, and Parker to the experience of black people as wanting to be assumed equal at the same time as wanting their centuries of oppression recognised. These two different contradictions can be difficult to keep in mind at the same time. Different sides of contradictions can easily get hidden in art therapy groups, sometimes between what is said and what is in the artwork, or in the many other dualities present.

In this chapter we have been working in a contradiction where, on the one hand, we are valuing the diversity in the different approaches on each side of the Atlantic while, on the other, our suggestion that contradictions should be exposed as such comes more from our own more psychoanalytically orientated tradition. Whilst all the projects we have selected for discussion are powerful interventions, and we recognise conflicts in all of them, our position is that those modes which privilege cognition, consciousness and directives are reflecting this same dominance in neoliberal ideology.

INTRODUCING PARTS TWO AND THREE

In the following chapters art therapy group work is described in which art therapists have grappled with the dynamics discussed here. Part Two is about the aftermath of the fire at Grenfell Tower. In Chapter Four, Susan Rudnik introduces Latimer Community Art Therapy (LCAT), a grassroots therapy project that sprung from the ashes of the fire, a preventable disaster in which 72 people lost their lives. She describes an ongoing relation of domination and resistance between the council and the community. Chapter Five describes a group for young people run in the community centre, which LCAT claimed back from the council. Beulah Lambert describes the dynamics that arose in the group when the young people made their voices heard in ways that created a lot of difficulty for the therapists. She is caught in a relation of power, which has meaning in both terms of adolescent development and in political activism. In Chapter Six, Holly Caldecourt describes her work in a primary school. Caldecourt had expected that the art therapy she provided to year one children would be for processing their experiences of the fire, however, the school had other ideas and asked her not to mention the fire. Caldecourt describes conflicting notions as to priorities, the school requiring education based on a restricted curriculum, measurements and targets whilst the art group process revealed that the children had other concerns, which the teachers found hard to hear.

Part Three is made up of contributions from art therapists working in institutions, community arts and in a refugee camp. In Chapter Seven, Mia Cavaliero describes difficulties running an art therapy group on an acute ward whilst the NHS is required to report patients who have unstable status to the Home Office for potential imprisonment and deportation. When senior staff enter the therapy space uninvited, Cavaliero asks herself if the group, as part of the acute ward, is a hostile environment or a place of safety. In Chapter Eight, Jessica Collier discusses the effects of political, social and misogynistic scapegoating of underprivileged women from the margins of society, and the way in which professionals and the prisoners themselves collude. Collier describes the impact of this on her running of art therapy groups. In Chapter Nine, Helen Omand discusses the conflict involved when an art therapeutic studio that has been supporting those with long-term mental health problems for decades faces drastic cuts. Where do therapy and protest meet? In this chapter the studio members tell us through presentations of their art work. In Chapter Ten, Emily Hollingsbee and Katie Miller travel to Greece to work in a refugee camp. They describe a tension between, on the one hand, offering a much-needed space for art and reflection, and on the other, realising that what they have to offer seems so minimal given the forces of oppression experienced by the refugees.

REFERENCES

Berman, H. (2017). Finding places and spaces for recognition: Applied art therapy training and practice in the mitigation against unthinking acts of violence. *Art Therapy OnLine,* 8(1), pp. 1–26.

Brooks, F. (1999). A Black Perspective on Art Therapy Training. In: Jones, J., Ward, C., Campbell, J., Liebmann, M., and Brooks, F. (eds), *Art Therapy, Race and Culture.* 1st ed., London and Philadelphia: Jessica Kingsley Publishers, pp. 275–286.

Canty, J. (2009). The key to being in the right mind. *International Journal of Art Therapy*, 14(1), pp. 11–16.

Coles, A. and Jury, H. (eds) (2020). *Art Therapy in Museums and Galleries: Reframing Practice*. London and Philadelphia: Jessica Kingsley Publishers.

Dalley, T. (2000). Back to the Future: Thinking about Theoretical Developments in Art Therapy. In: Gilroy, A. and McNeilly, G. (eds), *The Changing Shape of Art Therapy: New Developments in Theory and Practice*. London and Philadelphia: Jessica Kingsley Publishers, pp. 84–98.

Derrida, J. (1988). *Limited Inc.* S. Weber and J. Mehlman (trans.), G. Graff (ed.). Evanston: North Western University Press.

Dudley, J. (2011). Think Group: The median art psychotherapy group. *Art Therapy OnLine*, 2(1), pp. 1–26.

Estrella, K. (2011). Social Activism within Expressive Arts 'Therapy'. In: Levine, E. and Levine, S. (eds), *Art in Action: Expressive Arts Therapy and Social Change*. 1st ed, London and Philadelphia: Jessica Kingsley Publishers, pp. 42–52.

Foucault, M. (2000). *Essential Works of Foucault 1954–1984 Volume 2 Aesthetics*. R. Hurley and others (trans.), J.D. Faubion (ed.). London: Penguin Books.

Gilroy, A. and Skaife, S. (1997). Taking the pulse of american art therapy a report on the 27th annual conference of the american art therapy association, November 13th 17th, 1996, Philadelphia. *International Journal of Art Therapy: Inscape*, 2(2), pp. 57–64.

Gipson, L. (2018). Envisioning Black Women's Consciousness in Art Therapy. In: Talwar, S. (ed.), *Art Therapy for Social Justice: Radical Intersections*. 1st ed., London and New York: Routledge, pp. 96–120.

Heginworth, I.S. and Nash, G. (eds) (2019). *Environmental Arts Therapy: The Wild Frontiers of the Heart*. London: Routledge.

Hogan, S. (ed.) (1997). *Feminist Approaches to Art Therapy*. 1st ed., London: Psychology Press.

Hogan, S. (2009). The art therapy continuum: A useful tool for envisaging the diversity of practice in British art therapy. *International Journal of Art Therapy*, 14(1), pp. 29–37.

Hogan, S. (2015). *Art Therapy Theories: A Critical Introduction*. 1st ed., London and New York: Routledge.

Hogan, S. (2018). Gender Representation, Power, and Identity in Mental Health and Art Therapy. In: Hadley, B. and McDonald, D. (eds), *The Routledge Handbook of Disability Arts, Culture, and Media*. London and New York: Routledge, pp. 137–147.

Huss, E. (2009). 'A coat of many colors': Towards an integrative multilayered model of art therapy. *The Arts in Psychotherapy*, 36(3), pp. 154–160.

Jones, J., Ward, C., Campbell, J., Liebmann, M., and Brooks, F. (eds) (1999). *Art Therapy, Race and Culture*. 1st ed., London and Philadelphia: Jessica Kingsley Publishers.

Junge, M.B., Alvarez, J.F., Kellogg, A. and Volker, C. (1993). The art therapist as social activist: Reflections and visions. *Art Therapy*, 10(3), pp. 148–155.

Kapitan, L., Litell, M. and Torres, A. (2011). Creative art therapy in a community's participatory research and social transformation. *Art Therapy*, 28(2), pp. 64–73.

Kaplan, F. (2000). *Art, Science and Art Therapy: Repainting the Picture*. London and Philadelphia: Jessica Kingsley Publishers.

Layton, L. (2019). Transgenerational hauntings: Toward a social psychoanalysis and an ethic of dis-illusionment. *Psychoanalytic Dialogues*, 29(2), pp. 105–121.

LeBaron, M. (2011). Foreword. In: Levine, E.G. and Levine, S.K. (eds), *Art in Action: Expressive Arts Therapy and Social Change*. 1st ed., London and Philadelphia: Jessica Kingsley Publishers, pp. 9–18.

Levine, E. and Levine, S. (eds) (2011). *Art in Action: Expressive Arts Therapy and Social Change*. 1st ed., London and Philadelphia: Jessica Kingsley Publishers.

Levine, S.K. (1992). *Poiesis: The Language of Psychology and the Speech of the Soul*. Toronto: Palmerston Press/Jessica Kingsley Publishers.

Liebmann, M. (ed.) (1994). *Art Therapy with Offenders*. London: Jessica Kingsley Publishers.

Liebmann, M. (1997). Art therapy and empowerment in a women's self-help project. In: Hogan, S. (ed.), *Feminist Approaches to Art Therapy*. London and New York: Routledge, pp. 197–215.

Liebmann, M. and Ward, C. (1999). Art therapy and Jewish identity: Stories from Jewish art therapists. In: Campbell, J., Liebmann, M., Brooks, F., Jones, J. and Ward, C. (eds), *Art Therapy: Race and Culture*. London and Philadelphia: Jessica Kingsley Publishers, pp. 237–255.

Linnell, S. (2010). *Art Psychotherapy and Narrative Therapy: An Account of Practitioner Research*. Sharjah, United Arab Emirates: Bentham Science Publishers.

Lloyd, B. and Usiskin, M. (2020). Reimagining an emergency space: Practice innovation within a frontline art therapy project on the France–UK border at Calais. *International Journal of Art Therapy*, 25(3), pp. 132–142.

Maclagan, D. (2001). *Psychological Aesthetics: Painting, Feeling and Making Sense*. London and Philadelphia: Jessica Kingsley Publishers.

MacLeod, C. (2011). The Choreography of Absence. In: Levine, E. and Levine, S. (eds.), *Art in Action: Expressive Arts Therapy and Social Change*. 1st ed., London and Philadelphia: Jessica Kingsley Publishers, pp. 147–159.

McNiff, S. (1997). Art therapy: A spectrum of partnerships. *The Arts in Psychotherapy*, 24(1), pp. 37–44.

Melliar, P. and Bruhka, A. (2010). Round the clock: A therapist's and service user's perspective on the image outside art therapy. *International Journal of Art Therapy*, 15(1), pp. 4–12.

Moon, C. (1997). Art therapy: Creating the space we will live in. *The Arts in Psychotherapy*, 24(1), pp. 45–49.

'Najma', Kaczynski, T., Martyn, J. and Hollamby, E. (2021). Image, Narrative and Migration. In: West, J. (ed.), *Using Image and Narrative in Therapy for Trauma, Addiction and Recovery*. London and Philadelphia: Jessica Kingsley Publishers, pp. 282–297.

Olufemi, L. (2020). *Feminism, Interrupted: Disrupting Power*. London: Pluto Press.

Parker, P. (1978). For the White Person Who Wants to Know How to Be My Friend. In: Parker, P. *'Movement in Black', A Collection of Poetry*. Oakland, CA: Diana Press. Reprinted by Firebrand Books in 1989.

Schaverien, J. (1994). Analytical art psychotherapy: Further reflections on theory and practice, *Inscape*, 2, pp. 41–49.

Skaife, S. (2007). Working in Black and White: An Art Therapy Supervision Group. In: Schaverien, J. and Case, C. (eds), *Supervision of Art Therapy, a Theoretical and Practical Handbook*. London and New York: Routledge, pp. 139–152.

Skaife, S. (2013). Black and White: Applying Derrida to contradictory experiences in an art therapy group for victims of torture. *Group Analysis*, 46(3), pp. 256–271.

Skaife, S., Morris, L., Tipple, R. and Velada, D. (2020). The story of the camera, a case study of an art therapy large group. *Group Analysis*, *53*(1), pp. 37–59.

Talwar, S.K. (ed.) (2018). *Art Therapy for Social Justice: Radical Intersections*. 1st ed., New York and London: Routledge.

Tillet, S. and Tillet, S. (2018). 'You Want to Be Well?': Self-Care as a Black Feminist Intervention in Art Therapy. In: Talwar. S. (ed.), *Art Therapy for Social Justice*. London and New York: Routledge, pp. 123–143.

Waller, D. (2004). *Art Therapists: Pragmatic Rebels*. Goldsmiths College, University of London.

PART TWO

Grenfell

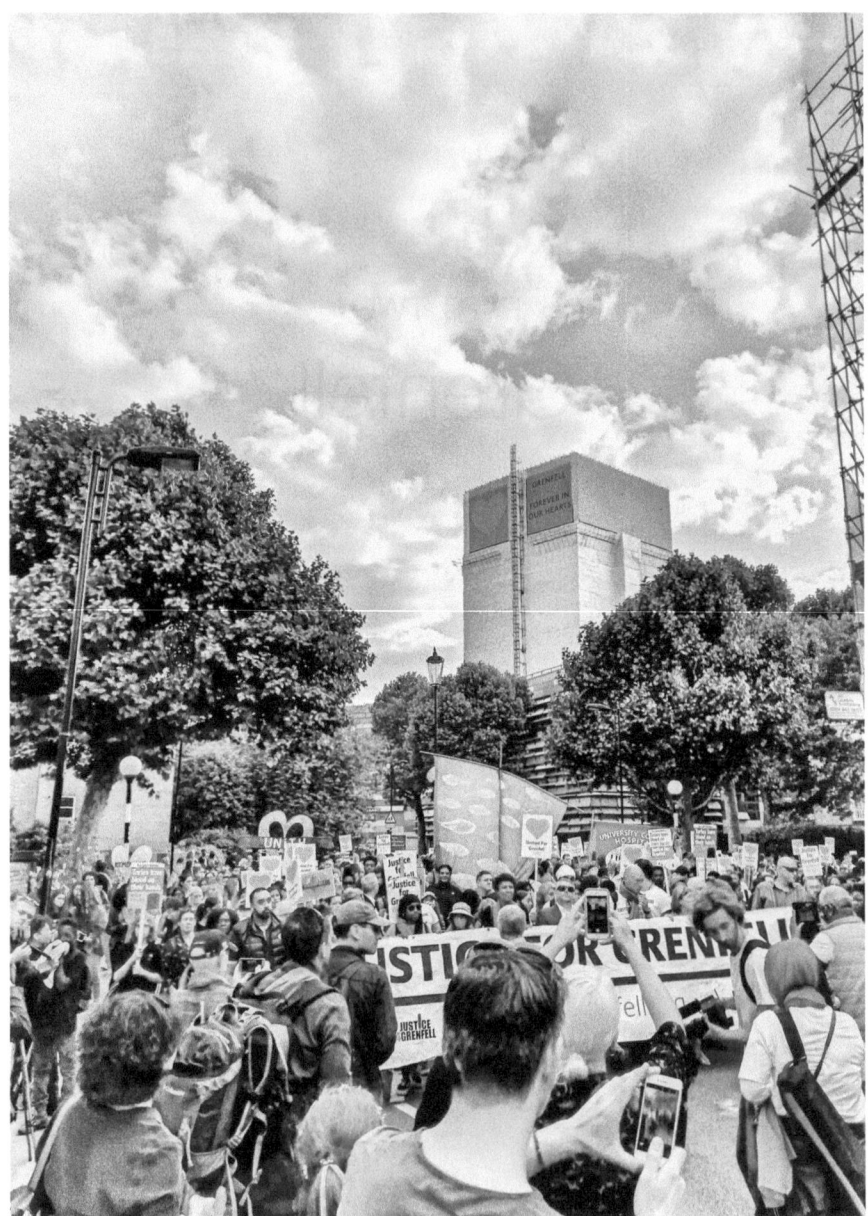

Figure P.2 *14th June 2018, Silent Walk for the 1st-year anniversary of the Grenfell fire. Photograph taken by @AndreiaSofiaPhotography.*

Monthly community-led 'Silent Walks' have taken place since the fire. The blackened tower was covered in a protective wrap in May 2018.

CHAPTER FOUR

Latimer Community Art Therapy
Developing from the grassroots after Grenfell

Susan Rudnik

DOI: 10.4324/9781003107408-6

INTRODUCTION

The Grenfell Tower fire of 14th June 2017, in which at least 72 people died, was the worst fire London has seen since the Second World War. The tower block, part of the Lancaster West Estate, is in one of the richest boroughs in London, the Royal Borough of Kensington and Chelsea (RBKC). RBKC houses royalty, celebrities and government officials, with houses in one exclusive street in the South selling for upwards of £35 million. In contrast, the North of the borough, where Grenfell stands, has a 38% child poverty rate and is dominated by social housing.

The blaze at Grenfell was sparked by a faulty tumble drier and fueled by the external cladding with disastrous consequence. Wrapped around the tower to fit for aesthetic purposes with the new school and leisure centre, the cladding ensured Grenfell 'did not look like a poor cousin' (Grenfell Tower Inquiry, 2021a, p. 34). The institutional indifference, managed decline and class contempt that led to the fire runs deep; RBKC chose to save £300,000 during the controversial refurbishment by cladding the tower in what is, by all extents and purposes, solidified petrol (Renwick, 2019).

The plans for the refurbishment of the tower were vehemently protested by residents, concerns being raised about access, fire escapes, sprinklers and much more. The stark warning from resident Edward Daffarn in his blog written in November 2016, which said that 'only a serious fire in a tower block would be the reason that those who wield power at the Kensington and Chelsea Tenant Management Organisation (KCTMO) would be found out and brought to justice' (Grenfell Tower Inquiry, 2021b, p. 3), formed part of his witness statement in the inquiry.

This chapter describes dynamics of power in relation to the development of Latimer Community Art Therapy (LCAT), from its beginnings immediately after the fire at Grenfell Tower, to three and a half years on. The development has been fraught with tension due to our dependence on RBKC, who could be considered responsible for the fire and who continue to hold power over us through their control of the space, the building and the finances. However, the community, too, has had power; the power to resist the dominant values of those by whom we are controlled and the power that comes from community solidarity in building an art therapy service by, and for, the community from the grassroots up. The chapter describes the experience of this from the inside.

RESISTANCE

North Kensington has a rich history of political resistance, occupation and revolt that spans decades before the fire. The Mangrove restaurant, hailed as a home from home to the Caribbean community, was unfairly targeted by police, but black activists stood up to power, took to the streets and fought for their space. Famously, the Mangrove 9 at the heart of this battle were taken to court but, eventually, acquitted of the charge of inciting a riot. The Free and Independent state of Frestonia, created by residents in 1977 to overthrow an eviction order to demolish their homes, forced the Greater London Council to rehome them together by renaming themselves with the same surname so that they would be considered as one family. This direct action gave them a voice in the plans and, ultimately, safe homes in the redevelopment where generations have flourished since. London's oldest adventure playground, Venture, built by children reclaiming a space to play on a derelict bomb site after World War 2, continues to this day. Finally, the Notting Hill Carnival, a vibrant annual event in the area, was born from resistance to the racially motivated killing of Kelso Cochrane in 1959. It inhabits our streets, asserting our rights to space and place. The very fabric of the community is made up of a culture of resistance. I have no doubt that this is in the social unconscious enabling LCAT and informing our thinking and action.

The two of us, Lucy Knight (a teacher) and myself, who have come to be the leaders of LCAT, are both connected to this resistance. Lucy has been familiar to the area all her life through family and through participation in carnival, and I am a local resident. I have come to think of my role as one of 'holding from the inside'; instilled in me is a sense that in the building of a strong art therapy community, immersion in locality is important.

THE BUILDING

The organic and grassroots evolution of LCAT began on Saturday 17th of June 2017 with the spontaneous making of an art therapy room in the Henry Dickens Community Centre. Henry Dickens is on the council estate in which I live and minutes from Grenfell Tower and the outreaching streets. Art therapists, who I brought in to help, met in my garden to think collectively about the work. Three years on, this same model is still in place. We have a core base at Henry Dickens, with two repurposed spaces made into art therapy rooms, an 'outreach' programme across fourteen schools and nurseries in North Kensington, and an adult service including a partnership with Age UK. The team consists of 15 art psychotherapists, 14 of which have been with LCAT since the beginning, developing and growing their practice as the organisation itself has developed.

The community centre, although given the term 'residents club house', was inaccessible to most residents, locked and underused for decades. Unlike other designated community buildings and spaces that were turned into respite centres, this space had not been opened as a place for support in the aftermath of the fire. The community took matters into their own hands and the building was broken open the morning after the fire by my neighbours on the estate, and taken back from the tight hold of KCTMO management. This was an unwitting political stand by two mothers who were unaccepting of the narrative put to them by the KCTMO that 'the keys were coming'. Donations were piling up and, tired of waiting, they took direct action, taking power where once they had none. That act essentially formed LCAT. We felt at once we could be in control of our own recovery and support those around us. Once neglected, our community centre was now lovingly cared for, windows and floors cleaned and scrubbed, we watched over the building like a baby.

In the days after the fire, after we had established art therapy groups and a space for the children to come after school, KCTMO suddenly changed the locks on the community centre, preventing access. This grabbed the attention of a reporter at the time and made it into a leading newspaper. 'The company responsible for managing Grenfell Tower has changed the locks on a community centre used to provide art therapy for children affected by the tragedy, stranding parents and children outside in the street when they came to seek help' (Graham-Harrison, 2017). We launched into action and collectively challenged this insidious move; within 24 hours the keys were returned to us.

Control of this building has remained controversial and complex. Reclaimed and rebuilt as our own, the symbolic importance of the community centre cannot be underestimated. It has provided the holding post disaster and still does. The fire not only destroyed lives and homes but it also destroyed our sense of safety, the concrete realisation that we were not safe in our homes rippled through the community, increasing anxiety and fear. Tucked away from street view, safe from journalists in the early weeks, the safety and warmth of the community centre was needed more than ever. It was used for meetings, therapeutic support, activism and, of course, a cup of tea. With this positive attachment to the building, a therapeutic process was able to take root and grow from there to the whole borough. This sense of community response was felt by us to be in stark contrast to that of RBKC and those given six figure salaries to manage our recovery.

MEETINGS

The question as to who held power was clear before the fire. We, the diverse working class of North Kensington, like many living in poor areas of London, were powerless. We could not stop nursery closures, gentrification and land grabbing. We certainly couldn't stop the fateful refurbishment of the Grenfell Tower. After the fire we suddenly appeared to have power – those in authority listened and gave time and attention to the groups and communities in the area. Lulled into a false sense of security we saved libraries, fought off estate regenerations and built services for ourselves, knowing all the while this was piecemeal for the sacrifice of 72 of our neighbours and the authority's catastrophic failure to care. However, the power held by RBKC never really shifted, and this was most evident in meetings at the time, which painfully highlighted the stark differences between 'us' and 'them'. The meetings were often volatile and challenging for us all. Mothers needed to attend to ensure they had their voices heard, and as a result the children would end up there, listening to adult conflict they had no control over. In response to this we decided to run children's groups at the meetings.

During one particular meeting held in the local social club, we sat with the children at the back of the hall whilst their parents and other adults faced RBKC officials, who were sat at the front in neat suits with pre-prepared answers. They were speaking about a desperate need for rehousing for families devastated by the fire. With each new platitude offered, and with the multitude of unanswered questions skillfully deflected, rage bubbled over. Meanwhile, the children at the back of the hall were drawing their own estate plans on large pieces of paper on the floor, putting in a helter-skelter, a sweet factory and a NASA space station; an antidote to what they were witnessing and perhaps an unconscious attempt to bring back life, aspirations and fun. One child made a snake from plasticine (see Figure 4.1), a 'highly poisonous snake', he announced. This somehow took on the appearance of the tower at the time, grey, lifeless with what looked like square windows along the body. This deadly creature remained on the table and we experienced it as a metaphor for the damage and poisonous venom present at the meeting in the form of the council, which had destroyed so much. Frequently, the children's groups seemed in a parallel process to the work of the adults. The children would decide on the rules and what was needed in their space just as the adults attempted to draw out new parameters for themselves. In another group, one child created a poster with what they wanted to use the time in the group for, with 'fun and good things' and 'noooo bad things' written in large letters. The drawing also depicted a person with a great deal of uncertainty in their face, seemingly stepping from turbulent waters to pastures new, symbolic of the precariousness of the desire for change in the community that both adults and children were asking for.

After some particularly volatile meetings we requested that the meetings be held in venues that were able to ensure a separate room for the

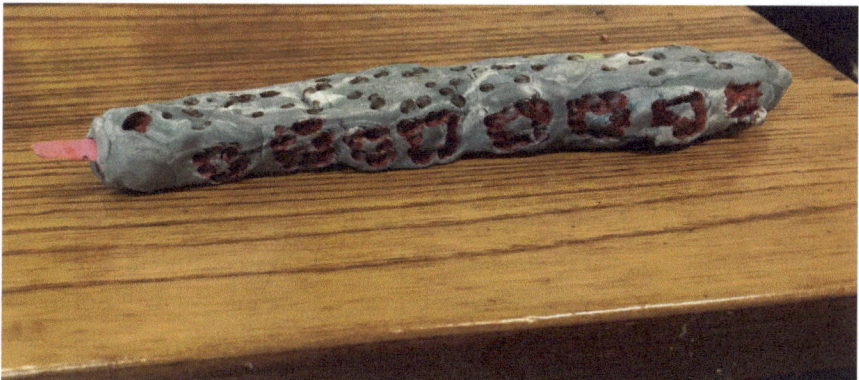

Figure 4.1 *'A highly poisonous snake'. Artwork made by a group member.*

children's groups. Despite this we could always hear the distant raised voices from the meetings. The children would, at times, exclaim proudly, 'that's my Mum I can hear', while at other times they would be more worried and need reassurance that all was okay. Mothers would come from the meetings, exhausted from battle, for a cuddle with their child and a tea break. As a local Mum, I often experienced a pull to want to be with the adults challenging the council, at the same time seeing the need to protect the children and give them the space to be heard and looked after. We named the children's groups 'safe spaces', intending to provide a sanctuary away from the difficult meetings. In hindsight, I recognise how much a safe space was needed in the community at the time, and our naming of this was not just for the children but also for us. The 'safe space' groups continued throughout the summer after the fire and carried on for over a year, providing consistency and a much-needed sanctuary for the children, as well as a space for their voices to be heard in their own way.

Gradually, local meetings became less frequent, official meetings slowly moved back to the RBKC town hall, away from the palpable rage of North Kensington to carpeted rooms in spaces in which we didn't belong. These scrutiny meetings became the new arena within which to challenge power and decisions about our recovery. We would come to question a panel of committee members, asking for answers after scrutinising policy, demanding change. At times, 'experts' in disaster recovery and trauma would be wheeled in to tell us about surviving post disaster, giving us a time scale for trauma recovery and instilling forced positivity that things would get better. This is all part of recovery they would say, it's ordinary for the state to get things wrong and for us to feel let down by them. Quite how wrong seemed to have eluded these experts. In July 2019, the Grenfell Recovery Scrutiny Committee meetings were scrapped by the council against vehement protest. Local activists and residents drowned out the last meeting, led in song by Niles Hailstones singing the classic Bob Marley protest song 'Small Axe', repeatedly stating, 'we will not betray the dead', as councillors shuffled out, heads bowed. A space to collectively and publicly challenge the council simply taken away. Instead, smaller conversations and meetings were offered and a return to documents being on the website should we care to look.

LCAT continues to meet with RBKC officials in charge of pots of money and pedalling an ever-evolving recovery plan, with ever-new frameworks, aims, consultations and agendas. Within these meetings it is painfully clear that LCAT's therapeutic model of care and a compassionate wish to help is at odds with the public sector business model approach.

CONFLICTING IDEAS ABOUT CARE AND RECOVERY

The ruling class in RBKC continue to assert authority and to control us, 'the workers', doing the work. This amounts to measuring, counting and an essentially reductionist way of quantifying the work and people's distress based on numbers and monetary values, a business model that suits a so-called evidence base with a manualised approach to mental health and trauma. This dehumanises and overlooks the importance of human connectedness, trusted relationships and working from experience. The chaos, mess and rabble of the working class continue to be seen as a problem that needs to be solved by control from middle-class management within RBKC, who seem unable to see that this authentic and creative process cannot simply be put into boxes and tidied up.

The very data that is asked for undermines the community approach that LCAT has and the ethos of our collective working and thinking; it individualises and commodifies the collective experience and removes the creative work that is the very fabric of LCAT. It also overlooks the multiplicity of ways that voices are heard and thought about within our work, particularly with children and adolescents. A truly authentic voice for the child is one which is led by them, in non-directive therapeutic work and community spaces that create space for play, art making and non-verbal communication. These allow the child's voice to come through in an authentic way for those that care to listen. In the early work of LCAT the voices of the children post disaster were embodied in the art making, chaos and mess in each community space and school. We thought they were unconsciously working with the imprint on them of the terrible reality that children just like them had experienced. This way of working is harder to commodify and churn out as data and, when we do, it loses all meaning. This uneasy fit of capturing the essence of therapeutic work and evidencing it is described by Dalal (2018) as akin to picking up soup with chopsticks – it simply cannot be grasped by those in charge unless fundamentally changed and distorted to become something else. LCAT has not been prepared to lumpify the soup to satisfy the bureaucracy within the local council, and therefore 'grasping' what we do eludes them.

The community continues to struggle to trust RBKC and, to date, the recovery plan has to be executed within a time-limited structure that is controlled by the very people that caused the disaster we are living through. Those in charge remain seemingly unable to accept the unknowns, mess and chaos of the work and to allow space for people to work through their experience. To truly allow this would mean to relinquish control and to trust a working-class community with power to help themselves.

AN ETHOS 'TAKES SHAPE'

No one could doubt that there were high levels of stress before the fire, but certainly since the fire, when people are unsafe in their homes, they are astronomically high. Blackwell (2019) talks about working with high levels of anxiety in uncertain times and the need to contain this enough to enable creativity. He warns that if the anxiety is not managed, it will 'escalate to the point where thought becomes increasingly difficult, if not impossible, and the system tips over into chaos or rigidifies into authoritarianism' (Blackwell, 2019, p. 71).

The containment of anxiety towards enabling creativity, then, has been one of our foremost aims. To this end, our structure enables space for thinking and development without micromanagement. The work is led by the individual within the context of the group – whether this is the child with her own idea of what craft activity to do in the community centre, or the clinician with a passion for working with a particular cohort of children given space to develop their practice. This flexible way of working allows LCAT to be built by all, much like the war-time adventure playground, Venture. The space is there and everyone contributes something to building the organisation.

Connections and conflicts within the work and between us, although not always easy to think about, are given space in monthly whole team supervision groups. The therapists are integrated into the community team through co-working and debriefs, as well as just ordinary connections and sharing of space. It is within this matrix that the unbearable anxiety has been able to be contained and the creative thinking needed for survival produced. The psychodynamic underpinning of LCAT affords an opportunity to think about the internal and external group processes and how they interlink with our clinical work and the unconscious defences, such as projection, alongside relational ways of working.

CONCLUSION

The air still feels thick in North Kensington, heavy with a weight that cannot be seen. You can still feel trapped here – everywhere you go the tower is visible, even at night, the green heart illuminated at the top visible from every corner of the borough. You are never away from it.

No way out, just round and round the misery of the system. Consultation upon consultation about how they can help us recover and forget and build resilience against a system that broke us, with no idea how it feels to be bringing up our children, knowing so concretely the system failed them and their friends and that nothing is safe anymore. Grenfell should have changed everything we say to each other. We know it has changed nothing, just us. We remain changed forever, never able to return to the lives we had before.

REFERENCES

Blackwell, D. (2019). Stability or Chaos, Authoritarianism or Dialogue; Towards a Matrix of Critical and Creative Thought at a Time of Uncertainty and Threat. In: Thornton, C. (ed.), *The Art and Science of Working Together: Practicing Group Analysis in Teams and Organisations*. 1st ed., London and New York: Routledge, pp. 67–75.

Dalal, F. (2018). *CBT: The Cognitive Behavioural Tsunami: Managerialism, Politics and the Corruptions of Science*. 1st ed., London and New York: Routledge.

Graham-Harrison, E. (2017). 'Company in charge of Grenfell Tower locks community out of therapy centre'. *The Guardian*, 29th June [online]. Available at: https://www.theguardian.com/uk-news/2017/jun/29/kctmo-company-in-charge-of-grenfell-tower-locks-community-out-of-therapy-centre [Accessed 27th June 2021].

Grenfell Tower Inquiry (2021a). Second witness statement of Edward Daffarn. Available at: https://assets.grenfelltowerinquiry.org.uk/IWS00002109_Phase%202%20witness%20statement%20of%20Edward%20Daffarn.pdf.

Grenfell Tower Inquiry (2021b). May 11, Day 128. Official Court Report; p. 1 Available at: https://assets.grenfelltowerinquiry.org.uk/documents/transcript/Transcript%2011%20May%202021.pdf.

Renwick, D. (2019). Organising on Mute. In: Bulley, D., Edkins, J. and El-Enany, N. (eds), *After Grenfell: Violence, Resistance and Response*. 1st ed., London: Pluto Press, pp. 19–46.

CHAPTER FIVE

'This is *Our* Group'

Art therapy with adolescents in the shadow of Grenfell

Beulah Lambert

DOI: 10.4324/9781003107408-7

The Grenfell Tower fire on 14 June 2017 devastated North Kensington, claiming at least 72 lives, leaving hundreds more homeless, bereaved and traumatised. As is coming to light in the ongoing public inquiry, a succession of deplorable decisions based on the needs of capital need rather than social need led to perilous living conditions in Grenfell Tower, and subsequently to the fire that took so many lives (Grenfell Action Group, 2017). As such, the most disheartening fact remains that the horrific event could have been avoided if not for the local authority's alleged contempt for residents and the corrupt multinational corporations that disregarded safety measures in order to make large financial profits. In the aftermath of the fire, the pre-existing disparity between the wealthy decision makers in power and working-class residents became further entrenched. Historical feelings of neglect were compounded by the council's reticence to provide support in the days and weeks after the fire, leaving the community to organise shelter and donations of food and clothing (Renwick, 2019). The experience of a top-down hostility permeated the psyches of residents across the borough: not only are the authorities untrustworthy, but they are directly implicated in this atrocity.

In this chapter I consider the social and emotional impacts of the fire on a group of young adolescents who live close to Grenfell Tower. I will do this by outlining the development of an open art therapy group that began days after the fire for children of all ages. I will describe the process of separating the group into different spaces for older and younger children in response to requests from the adolescents. This division became a source of conflict within the adolescent group, as will be explored. I look at their resistance towards therapeutic boundaries in relation to their journey into adolescence, experiences of authority following the fire and pre-existing deprivation. Equally, I aim to highlight how social class struggles and wealth disparities, which were exposed and exacerbated by the avoidable tragedy, emerged in the group within the context of such conflicts within the community.

THE EARLY SERVICE

Three days after the fire Susan Rudnik, a resident on the Henry Dickens (HD) social housing estate and an art therapist, set up a therapeutic space in the HD Community Centre close to Grenfell Tower. I vividly remember my journey to the community centre just days after the disaster, as the impact of the fire was inescapable. Police cordons still in place, I passed hundreds of posters of 'missing' children and adults, and boxes of donations piled high. The tower, standing in plain sight, eerily appeared around every corner, and was visible for miles around. Tributes to those lost, graffiti demanding justice and anti-establishment slogans berating the council decorated the streets. I felt highly anxious about the traumatic state the children might be in and hesitant about my ability to facilitate art therapy groups amongst the disarray I anticipated. On arriving at the community centre, I learnt that most of the children who were coming into the centre lived on the HD estate and were bereaved, having lost teachers, friends and neighbours. Others had witnessed the horror of the fire whilst looking on helplessly from their homes, and all had overheard graphic stories and experienced the grief felt amongst their community. Inside the therapy room it felt as if we were operating an emotional A&E, the space spilling over with children and adolescents aged between two to fourteen years old, expressing their distress through jumbled up words and messy artworks. All we could do at this point was offer a holding space for these children whose sense of safety had been unreservedly shattered. At this point, 'the ordinary boundaries we hold so dear in therapy seemed useless' (Rudnik, 2018, p. 4), as it felt as if the community needed something beyond any possible theory or therapeutic framework. For months the door to the art therapy room remained open, welcoming children and their parents to drop into the daily three-hour groups. Although unusual for children's therapy groups, maintaining an open-group model seemed most appropriate. The children's ability to choose when to attend the groups and how long to remain in them seemed to enable trust and helped nurture a culture of care and containment, crucial when the community were understandably dubious about trusting professionals. Artwork was either left unnamed and unclaimed or taken home. We had little background on the children who simply appeared in our service, some attending daily and others only once. Gradually, discussions with parents gave us snippets of information, 'he lost his best friend', 'we can't sleep', 'she saw the fire and heard the screaming'.

In the groups, the creation of artwork evidently served a vital function in terms of expression and containment. However, due to the busy flurry of activity given the high numbers of children attending, it often felt impossible to reflect upon what these artworks represented, let alone witness them as they were being created. It seemed that the children were equally unable to consciously connect with what they were creating, but at the end of each group I was taken aback by the sheer quantity of artworks and the strong emotions they evoked in me. I started to notice ash-like mixtures, images of charred towers, and tower-like constructions that had been created and destroyed (Figure 5.1). I experienced their artworks as imbued with life and emotion that simply could not be

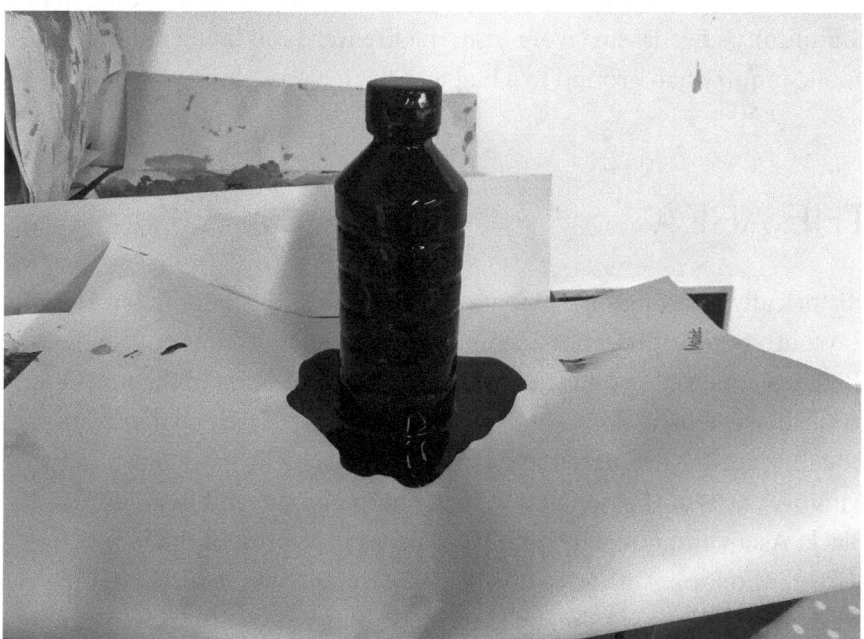

Figure 5.1 '... ash-like mixture'. Artwork made by a group member.

articulated in words. In supervision I was able to more clearly view the highly messy artworks as holding the children's distress and enabling the evacuation of the horror and chaos that was too disturbing to internalise. There was an apparent contradiction between the often gloopy, smelly mixtures and their status as highly precious items that the children were desperate to keep safe. I now realise the art materials not only served a containing function for the children, but also for us therapists. At a highly unpredictable and challenging time, these concoctions enabled us to tolerate and gradually reflect upon the children's strong projections of pain and suffering. Perhaps this was because they could be held inside physical containers and not solely in our minds.

After six months of working with children of all ages together, those moving onto secondary school started expressing frustration at the younger ones' immaturity, saying they needed to discuss issues such as puberty, discrimination and their sexuality. As such, we felt it necessary to provide a separate therapeutic group for the adolescents on a weekly basis. Perhaps our desire to meet their needs and alter the group was contextualised by the fact that the authorities were not responding to the community's needs: survivors from the fire were still living in hotels, the public inquiry had ground to a halt and justice was a long way off.

THE AREA

Historically, Kensington is known for its social and economic divide, with the south of the borough made up of embassies, museums and some of the most expensive properties in the country, and parts of the north home to various extensive social housing estates characterised by deprivation. Equally, North Kensington has a highly ethnically diverse community, with over 50% of the population being born abroad, and twice as many Black, Asian and minority ethnic groups as in the rest of the borough (Greater London Authority, 2017). This diversity was reflected in our art therapy clients, with many families coming from countries including Morocco, Somalia and the Caribbean. My co-therapist and I, both of mixed Black Caribbean and White British heritage, also mirrored this racial diversity, a supposed rarity within a context where the majority of therapists are white (Lumpkin, 1998, Holland, 2011).

From discussions with community members I understood that following the fire, class, wealth and race disparities were intensified; the community felt that the privileged middle- and upper-class white council officials had overlooked the needs of working-class, largely non-white, residents of the tower by authorising its inadequate refurbishment. Despite not living in the community myself, I instantly felt very much at home there, perhaps drawing on my own experiences of being racially different from the majority of the UK as a mixed-race person. At the time, I wondered to what extent my ethnicity might represent a possibility of understanding experiences of discrimination. Perhaps I had a fantasy I might be accepted by the community due to the shared experience of being a non-white 'other'. Nonetheless, I was also very aware that social class differences existed between the adolescents and me, with them living on a housing estate and myself a middle-class professional.

THE ADOLESCENT GROUP

Despite the requests from the adolescents for a separate therapeutic space, on starting the group their response became highly resistant. They complained that the time and day were wrong, and they did not like that the group was now exclusive to their age group. In fact, the first five sessions in which I was the only therapist felt like absolute chaos. Younger siblings were invited in, as if in protest, and instructed not to leave, while group members proclaimed, 'I want it to be like before', 'this is our group, we want them to stay'. When I tried to speak, they shouted over me. It felt as though they were attempting to exert power and control over me by shutting me out entirely. Extremely messy artworks were made frantically, with paint and water spilling onto the floor, and it felt impossible to keep up with them. Their constant running in and out of the room and refusal to comply with the new boundary of who was permitted in the group left me feeling out of control. I also felt an overpowering sense of danger, as if their uncontained messy artworks would continue to spill out and I might be drowned by the intensity of their projections. Nonetheless, however difficult I found it to tolerate the mess and the boundary pushing, I strongly believed that these adolescents needed a space to externalise their feelings. But I realised that I needed someone to share this with, and so I sought the support of a co-therapist, Charlotte Daley. I informed the group that another art therapist would be joining me in running the group in session six. I tried to think with them about how they felt about her arrival, to which they responded, 'does it look like we care?' Following their chaotic behaviour in the previous sessions I wondered if they would experience Charlotte's presence as indicative of my inability to 'cope' with them. Equally, considering their expression of ownership of the space, might they feel she was an intruder in their group?

In our first session together Charlotte and I found ourselves alone in the room. A period of minimal attendance continued for a number of weeks. I felt a sense of humiliation that I had sought assistance with this 'challenging group' and now no one was attending. Gradually, group members experimented with coming in. On entering, they expressed anger, shouting, 'this is our group', 'we don't know Charlotte'. Various liquidy artworks were created that spilled off the tables; they then exited. With our persistence in holding the group despite the low attendance, after six weeks a consistent group of young people started to come weekly. Recycled containers holding murky mixtures made previously and cardboard boxes were reclaimed and personalised. Discussions followed regarding their teachers' neglectful and discriminatory attitudes, 'they are terrible', 'they just do it for the money'. We asked if they thought that we were uncaring too and not good enough, like these teachers. Despite their responding, 'shut up, are we talking to you?', this suggestion enabled them to ask us questions, 'do you get paid?', 'what qualifications do you have?'. Week after week group members created messy artworks, regularly using up entire bottles of paint and then angrily demanding more. Regardless of our attempts to think with them about this, and our encouragement to try other art materials that were in plentiful supply, they were unable to reflect upon this insatiable desire for paint. We commented that perhaps the free-flowing nature of the paint helped release their feelings, which was met with, 'stop talking like that, we aren't mental'. Given the speed at which paint was used up, we had already decided we would only replenish the art materials once a month, as we worried the funds to get more would run out. We explained that we shared the resources with everyone in the community centre and wanted to ensure we would have enough for this group to run long-term. However, the group knew that for the time being we had a well-stocked art cupboard, and said, 'it's not fair', 'we know you have so many art materials, just give us some'. I felt extremely cruel and withholding as if I was unfairly depriving them, and I was uncomfortable with the position of power I found myself in. The group also regularly demanded to take their artwork home, sometimes removing it despite, or perhaps because of, our requests for them not to. Other times, artworks would be disposed of, poured down the drain or smeared across tables as if they lacked any importance at all. We attempted to explain that we wanted to keep their artwork safely in the centre as it potentially represented their very difficult feelings that we wanted to hold for them, and to gradually help them process. We said that we thought their artwork was important and understood their fear that we might not be able to keep them, or their creations, safe. Our comments were met with, 'shut up', 'I don't want to hear your ugly voice'. Equally, our thinking about the disposal of artwork in terms of getting rid of unwanted feelings was experienced as infuriating, further escalating challenging behaviours.

After six months, a period of settling emerged in the group – two-dimensional artworks were created and kept within folders, and liquids remained within containers. Conversations about the group members' personal lives entered the group and it felt as if trust was emerging. It still felt difficult to trace their experiences of the fire, as there was a sense of their remembering and forgetting, of wanting and not wanting to discuss it. However, on approaching the one-year anniversary this seemed to shift. Multiple memorial events were scheduled and media crews started popping up around the vicinity of the tower. In the community, there was growing frustration with the lack of developments in the public inquiry, along with fears that justice would not be achieved due to suspicions about corruption and attempts to conceal evidence. Sensing the community's heaviness and collective anxiety, we gently opened up space in the group to think about what feelings the anniversary might bring up. We were overwhelmed by emotions and graphic descriptions: anger and frustration towards the council, teary recollections of what they witnessed, nightmare-like thoughts of people trapped inside the tower surrounded by corpses, and moving stories of peers who had died. We spoke about the spilling of paints in previous sessions as linked to the expression of difficult feelings related to the fire itself. This seemed to encourage greater verbal expression of feelings as conversations about the loss of grandparents and fears about death emerged. We spoke about how difficult the anniversary might be, not only in terms of Grenfell, but also in triggering other experiences of loss.

The week of the anniversary we had a particularly notable group. Multiple new members joined and one young person spent time creating a large banner that read 'JUSTICE FOR GRENFELL', referencing the community's campaign for justice. The creator of this piece announced that it would be 'permanently displayed on the wall as a reminder of why we are here'. We commented on the power and importance of the piece and then asked the group their thoughts on it being displayed, to which they responded, 'I don't care', 'why can't she put her artwork up?' We tried to think about what impact this artwork might have on others who used the room and suggested that she only display the artwork for the duration of the group that day. She shouted, 'you don't care about justice! What's the point of making it if no one will see it?' I wondered if she experienced our suggestion as a personal rejection as well as an indication that we were not in solidarity with the community's campaign for justice. Suddenly the group spun out of control. Some group members stormed about the room shouting angrily, others placed multiple paint-covered hands on the windows, and whole tables became canvases for artwork as an entire bottle of black paint was squirted and spread (Figure 5.2). I had strong feelings of uselessness and fear that their anger would overwhelm us all. It felt incredibly challenging to think about what was being communicated and to not respond by stopping the group or simply becoming strict boundary enforcers. Struggling to let our voice be heard above the commotion, we commented that although permanent marks may not be made in the room, we were trying to understand what they were trying to tell us. We suggested that perhaps they were expressing their feelings about the anniversary, the lack of justice following the fire and the incredible unfairness of our boundaries about what they could and could not do. This only seemed to escalate their anger as they shouted, 'shut up, stop talking about feelings'. At this point, one group member attempted to jump out of the ground floor window onto the concrete some metres below. I blocked the window, insisting this was unsafe, which was met with fury. Everyone suddenly left, smearing paint across the door and walls as they went.

Grateful I was not alone in the messy room, I reflected with Charlotte on what had just occurred. We wondered if the group had experienced their anger as overwhelming, characterised by the sudden desire to leave. The black paint that covered the entire table was reminiscent of the burnt tower. We thought about how my attempt to ensure safety by prohibiting an exit from the window might have been experienced as a

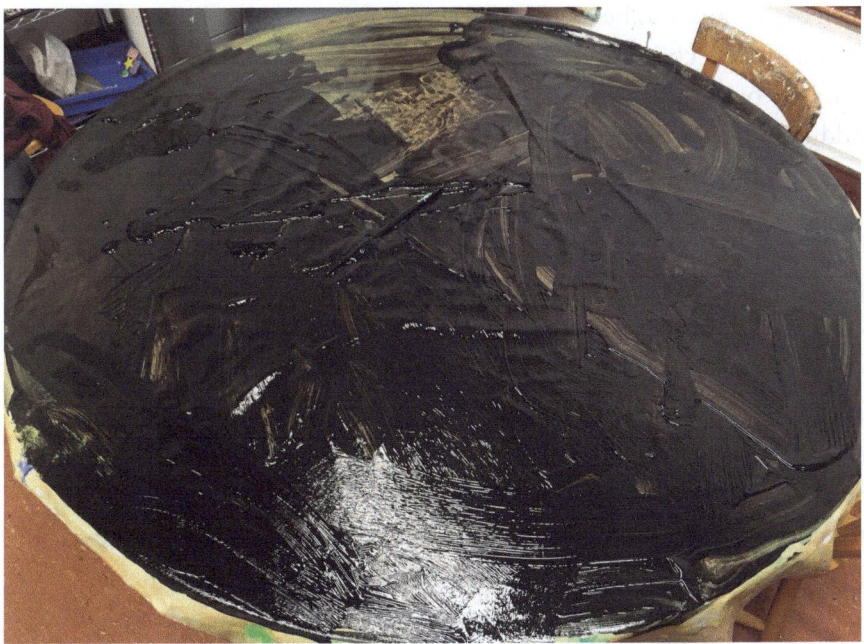

Figure 5.2 *'Black paint spread across the whole table.' Artwork made by the group.*

cruel entrapment rather than an act of care. I could not help but think of Grenfell Tower residents being told to stay put by the authorities, and how dangerous and fatal this advice had been. Equally, the desire to jump out of the window and the painty handprints felt highly disturbing. They were evocative of residents desperately banging at windows while the flames roared behind them, and of those who tragically jumped from the tower to escape the inferno within.

THE SEPARATION OF THE ADOLESCENT GROUP

As has been explored, I regularly had strong feelings of incompetence and even despair throughout this piece of work. On starting the group, I was confused by the adolescents' resistance as I felt that I was responding positively to their requests. On reflection, separating the therapy groups quite possibly painfully accentuated their pre-existing feelings. Comments such as, 'I want it to be like before' exposed a mourning linked to multiple losses: of their childhood brought about by the onset of puberty, of the vibrancy of their community before the fire, and of those who died. Additionally, the sense of exclusion felt palpable, younger children not being permitted in the group represented exclusivity, evocative of the division in the borough between rich and poor. Perhaps my feeling of not being good enough symbolised the political climate in the community at the time. Nothing was good enough; it was all a big mess. No amount of donations or offers of emotional support can remove the horror of the fire. The tower, uncovered for almost a year, like a charred still-standing corpse, served as a potent reminder of how utterly horrific everything was. As such, the adolescents' anger at our decision to limit the art materials signified more than an urge for paint. It appeared to be connected to their experiences of systematic socio-economic failings, characterised by their community's historic deprivation and neglect. I wonder if our class differences enhanced this – was there envy about our access to materials and our power to withhold or allocate resources as middle-class professionals? Perhaps this mirrored the council's decisions to restrict money in the refurbishment of Grenfell Tower and limit support following the fire. My feelings of inadequacy seemed inherently linked to the group's own sense of being undervalued as adolescent and working class. As trust in professionals had been violently ruptured, comments such as, 'this is our group', extended well beyond the therapeutic space, as if to say, 'this is our estate, who are you to tell us what we can and cannot do here?' I wonder who we represented in the transference: were we the teachers who were 'only doing it for the money'? Or, irrespective of our race, as paid professionals were we the local authority officials who could not identify with the community's experiences of social struggle? Undoubtedly, whomever we represented, we were experienced as powerful figures of authority.

BOUNDARIES

Dizadji, in Blackwell and Dizadji (2016), argues that highly flexible boundaries are imperative when working with communities suffering from deprivation and trauma. She advocates for therapists' active engagement and merging in with communities. Elsewhere, Blackwell (2015) states that disadvantaged inner-city youth often require a more political approach as a result of race and class inequalities. Nonetheless, there is no theoretical blueprint of working with a disaster such as Grenfell. Despite trying to employ a flexible approach, it often felt as if we could not get things right and that we were on the edge of a precipice of uncontainable chaos. Given that we had arrived on the housing estate in the midst of community-wide disarray, this was not entirely surprising. However, such feelings evoked countertransference responses of fear. I wonder how this fear influenced our understanding of the group's needs and what boundaries were appropriate. Discussions between Charlotte and myself often revolved around the topic of safety: what minimal boundaries were imperative to keep the adolescents safe, how far were we safely able to tolerate their pushing these boundaries? Now we ask on reflection, who should have decided the relevant therapeutic confines within this community owned space? Whose group was it?

Despite how disordered the group felt, perhaps we could have attempted a more collaborative approach in deciding the boundaries. Or did they indeed need us to instigate boundaries to have something tangible to direct their anger towards? Maybe our preoccupation with safety was contextualised by a desire to distance ourselves from the local authority's failings in regards to safety. Paradoxically, no matter how liberal our approach, any boundaries we implemented may have been perceived to mirror the authorities that were the source of much rage within the community. What did our professionalism and boundaries represent to the adolescents? Within the context of the fire, our boundaries must have represented an oppressive force that was inconsiderate of their needs. Our job seemed an impossible balancing act: enabling space for the expression of anger, political protest and resistance whilst also providing enough containment via the very boundaries that made them angry. This impossibility manifested in what felt like a struggle between 'us' and 'them', evocative of class tensions between the community and the council. For example, did the group remove their artwork from the room because we asked them not to? Equally, I had understood the disposal of artwork as a getting rid of painful experiences that were too difficult to think about. However, much like taking their artwork, I wonder if it also encompassed a resistance to our authority. Perhaps their artwork was the sole thing they had control over and so they were even willing to destroy it for empowerment.

THE ARTWORK

Week after week, messy artworks were created and spread around the room. The volume of these artworks was a powerful reminder of the inescapability of their trauma, much like the charred tower is a constant reminder of the community's utter devastation. The repetitiveness of the mess seemed more than the externalising or projecting of feelings. It appeared the group wanted concrete indications that we could sit in the mess with them, and perhaps they were exploring if we, like other professionals, would simply remain apart, untouched by them. Aldridge (1998) and O'Brien (2004) explore extensive mess making in art therapy with children and young people who have experienced deprivation and trauma. Both authors highlight the internal difficulties arising from such issues that appear in the artwork as mess. However, neither considers how the therapist's class position plays out in the dynamic between client and therapist and may manifest in the artwork. Through their artwork, the adolescents brought us, and our positions as professionals, into the work. Their highly messy artworks repeatedly covered and stained our clothes, physically immersing and covering us in their suffering. Seemingly, to be trusted we had to allow ourselves to be touched by their trauma and 'merge in' with them (Blackwell and Dizadji, 2016), as symbolised by our literally being covered by their mess. It seemed they perceived the language of therapy as representative of middle-class values and rhetoric that felt irrelevant and oppressive. As such, I wonder if the paint on our clothes was also a communication of what these garments represented in terms of our being middle-class professionals, not from the area, who were getting paid for our work with them. With this in mind, their artwork could be viewed as more than projective or embodied, as an outpouring of emotion also linked to who we were in relation to them.

ADOLESCENCE AND RESISTANCE

I often felt we were far from engaging in any 'real' therapeutic work, as it seemed we were simply surviving the adolescents' unprocessed rage and resistance towards us. In part, such feelings seemed inherently linked to their journey into adolescence. As is well known, it is not uncommon for adolescents to display behaviour to resist and challenge authority. Waddell (2018) outlines that in the search for the sense of self, adolescents often rebel against parental figures, especially those felt to be authoritarian. Waddell also explores the particularly destabilising effect of adverse external events during this period. On reflection, actions within the group extended beyond adolescent acting out, and could be understood as politically motivated and in response to what was occurring around them. Blackwell's (2015) analysis of the 2011 London Riots seems relevant here. Contrasting media depictions that focused on the mass looting, violence and arson of young delinquents, Blackwell understands their response in terms of 'significant communications, intelligible within the various contexts within which they can be located' (2015, p. 104). Not unlike North Kensington, he describes these contexts as characterised by histories of oppression, deprivation and class and race struggles. Although at times we felt the adolescents were unconsciously acting out and pushing boundaries, with Blackwell's view in mind, one can clearly comprehend their rage as justified political protest. Of course the young people were angry. Seventy-two people, including 18 children, had died because they had been systematically failed and neglected by the very authorities that were meant to keep them safe. The groups' protesting behaviour was informed by what they were learning from their community's response to the tragedy in terms of socially active resistance. Through the formation of organisations campaigning for justice, influencing the process of the public inquiry, and holding silent walks on the 14th of every month, the community was resisting the authorities that had historically sought to silence them (Tuitt, 2019). However slow and inadequate the response, the adults who are campaigning for justice have access to formal avenues to express their sentiments and can thus attempt to hold the authorities to account, whereas the young people had no such arena. Perhaps the group provided a space to explore their own forms of political action by expressing and working through their feelings towards us as figures of authority. Such behaviour may have been the only way the group could begin communicating their experiences: namely, their community's pre-existing deprivation and class struggles, the trauma and inequality of the fire, and all the challenges of entering adolescence during this tumultuous time. The group was exceedingly challenging at times, but what I came to realise was that the group's resistance to our boundaries had become an integral part of the therapy itself. And this was extremely important. Living in a community that had been so tragically violated and failed, it felt imperative that the young people protest as a matter of survival. As the adolescents seemed unified in their challenges to our authority, I wonder if the group offered the members the opportunity for a socially active and cohesive identity, which seemed increasingly important at a time of such chaos and grief.

At the time of writing this group is still running.

REFERENCES

Aldridge, F. (1998). Chocolate or shit: Aesthetics and cultural poverty in art therapy with children. *Inscape*, 3(1), pp. 2–9.

Blackwell, D. (2015). Reading the riots London 2011: Local revolt and global protest. *Psychotherapy and Politics International*, 13(2), pp. 102–114.

Blackwell, D. and Dizadji, F. (2016). Demonised, blamed, negated, and disappeared: The victimisation of the poor in the globalised economy. *Psychotherapy and Politics International*, 14(1), pp. 5–16.

Greater London Authority (2017). London Area Profiles [website]. Available at: https://data.london.gov.uk/london-area-profiles/ [Accessed 7th October 2018].

Grenfell Action Group (2017). Grenfell Tower – The KCTMO Culture Of Negligence, 19th June [blog]. Available at: https://grenfellactiongroup.wordpress.com/2017/06/19/grenfell-tower-the-kctmo-culture-of-negligence/ [Accessed 22nd October 2018].

Holland, S. (2011). Psychotherapy, Oppression and Social Action: Gender Race and Class in Black Women's Depression. In: Perelberg, R. and Miller, A. (eds), *Gender and Power in Families*. 1st ed., London: Karnac Books, pp. 256–269.

Lumpkin, C. (1998). We Wear the Masks: A Study of Black Art Therapy Students. In: Hiscox, A. and Calisch, A. (eds), *Tapestry of Cultural Issues in Art Therapy*. 1st ed., London: Jessica Kingsley Publishers, pp. 219–228.

O'Brien, F. (2004). The making of mess in art therapy: Attachment, trauma and the brain. *Inscape*, 9(1), pp. 2–13.

Renwick, D. (2019). Organising on Mute. In: Bulley, D., Edkins, J. and El-Enany, N. (eds), *After Grenfell: Violence, Resistance and Response*. 1st ed, London: Pluto Press, pp. 19–46.

Rudnik, S. (2018). Out of the darkness: A community led art psychotherapy response to the Grenfell Tower fire. *Art Therapy OnLine*, 9(1), pp. 2–9.

Tuitt, P. (2019). Law, Justice and the Public Inquiry into the Grenfell Tower Fire. In: Bulley, D., Edkins, J. and El-Enany, N. (eds), *After Grenfell: Violence, Resistance and Response*. London: Pluto Press, pp. 119–129.

Waddell, M. (2018). *On Adolescence*. London: Karnac.

CHAPTER SIX

Don't go out *that* door

The pressure on a school to perform/conform whilst its community faces the aftermath of a disaster

Holly Caldecourt

DOI: 10.4324/9781003107408-8

I learnt of the fire at Grenfell Tower, which started in the early hours of 14th June 2017, when I woke that morning and, as usual, turned on the radio. Hearing about the fire within a residential tower block in West London did not prepare me for the images of complete devastation I saw soon after. A couple of weeks later I had begun working for Latimer Community Art Therapy (LCAT). I arrived in North Kensington, not unfamiliar to the area, but as an outsider to the community. In the streets, tributes and posters for the missing adorned walls and railings; the impact of this was palpable.

In this chapter I am going to describe an art therapy group in a North Kensington primary school for a class of year one children whose behaviour was seen by teachers to be 'needy' and 'disruptive'. I understood the children's behaviour to be a communication about the chaos around them and our intention for the therapy was to create a space in which to act as witnesses to the children's stories in relation to the fire, and to attempt to make sense of them together in a group. However, the school management seemed to want the disruptive behaviour to be dealt with as quickly as possible in order that the children get on with the formalised national curriculum.

The referral from the school came to LCAT in the late autumn term of 2017, almost six months following the fire. On receipt, Alice, my co-therapist, and I met with the Special Educational Needs Coordinator (SENCo) who reported, 'the children in the class are not getting along, it's as if they just don't like each other'. The SENCo explained that they had exhausted attempts to support the class teacher and teaching assistant with the children's needs. On hearing that their usual strategies of 'CBT zones of regulation' and behaviour policies had not managed to settle the children, I felt as if the request for an art psychotherapy intervention might be a last resort.

We arranged for a class observation with their class teacher and their teaching assistant (TA). The children were a rich mix of ethnicities, with a high proportion of families with multiple and complex needs, including children in temporary accommodation as a result of the fire. After observing a lesson, we understood why the school had described the children as 'needy'; they seemed to be constantly seeking reassurance from their teachers. Coming in from the playground, some children were in tears, which took time and attention from the staff to resolve. Whilst each altercation was being dealt with in a calm and nurturing manner, the other children began to fight and bicker. With these constant interruptions progress in the lesson was slow, and soon almost everyone had lost focus on what was being taught.

After the observation the teacher informed us that one of the children in the class had died in the fire. I was surprised that this had not been named in the referral. We were also told that several parents were entering the classroom at the end of the day upset over minor incidents that had often gone unnoticed in the playground. Relationships seemed strained between the school and parents of children in the class, and amongst the parents themselves.

Shortly before the work was to begin, Alice and I met with the class teacher and senior leadership. The Head made a request that we did not talk about the fire or the bereavement in the group to avoid upsetting the children. This was a pivotal moment between us and the school; we wondered if they would want us to deliver the group at all if we contested this, so with hesitation, we agreed. When we requested that the group last at least the duration of the spring term, the management team seemed nervous and noncommittal. I felt that we had been brought in with the unspoken expectation that we were to provide a solution, to deliver an intervention that would make the distress and chaos go away immediately, otherwise it was us, the therapists, who were expendable.

We left the meeting wondering how we were going to comply with the request not to speak of the fire; the charred remains of the tower were visible from windows within the school and from the playground; the effects of the disaster seemed to be everywhere I looked. The request felt like a burden that would only confuse the work.

Influenced by Dean Reddick's (2008) whole class intervention, Alice and I decided to structure the group art making around a theme of 'creatures'. We hoped the theme would be both vague enough to encompass a wide response from the children as well as encourage group cohesion. We thought that the children might bring their stories of the fire to the work through the theme and, in doing so, create an opportunity to think about

their experiences together as a group. This felt like a suitable way to adapt to
the school's request. We began the group in January 2018 without knowing
how long it could go on for. We planned to assess the work with the
management after four sessions in order to get agreement for it to continue.

THE FIRST FOUR GROUP SESSIONS

Initially we started in the children's classroom with the whole class
altogether, including the teacher and assistant. To begin the first session,
Alice and I had rearranged the classroom, grouping together some of
the tables and laying out materials in the middle of them. We introduced
ourselves to the children as art therapists, with the acknowledgement
that we were aware of some difficulties they had suffered. One child
interrupted and shouted out that there had been a 'big fire'. This gave
me a huge sense of relief – the fire had been named, which we read as
an indication that the children needed to talk about it. While we were
tempted to give space for the children to discuss the fire there and then,
the school's concerns made it feel rebellious to do so. So we decided to
stick to our plan, setting the theme and saying to the group that they
could use the art materials how they wished and we would come back
together afterwards to look at their work together.

The children dispersed quickly into a flurry of activity, some choosing to
sit at the tables while others worked on the floor, either independently
or in pairs, and some moved freely around the room. What began with
delight soon turned into chaos and conflict, with fights breaking out
over the emptied and scattered materials. It became hard to think, with
my attention pulled in different directions as I heard my name called
by children across the room. A couple of quieter children struggled to
know what to do at all and looked to their teacher for direction; they
ended up copying the teacher's image of a bird. There seemed to be
admiration for the teacher as well as a desire to be close to her. The
artworks varied greatly from lions to fish, to butterflies and rainbows. On
closer inspection, a common depiction of a tower ran through several
images. One image included a clearly drawn tower block, standing alone

in a seemingly foreign landscape. Another contained a large rectangular rainbow as if framing an invisible tower, presenting the absence of what could not be spoken of in the space beneath it (Figure 6.1).

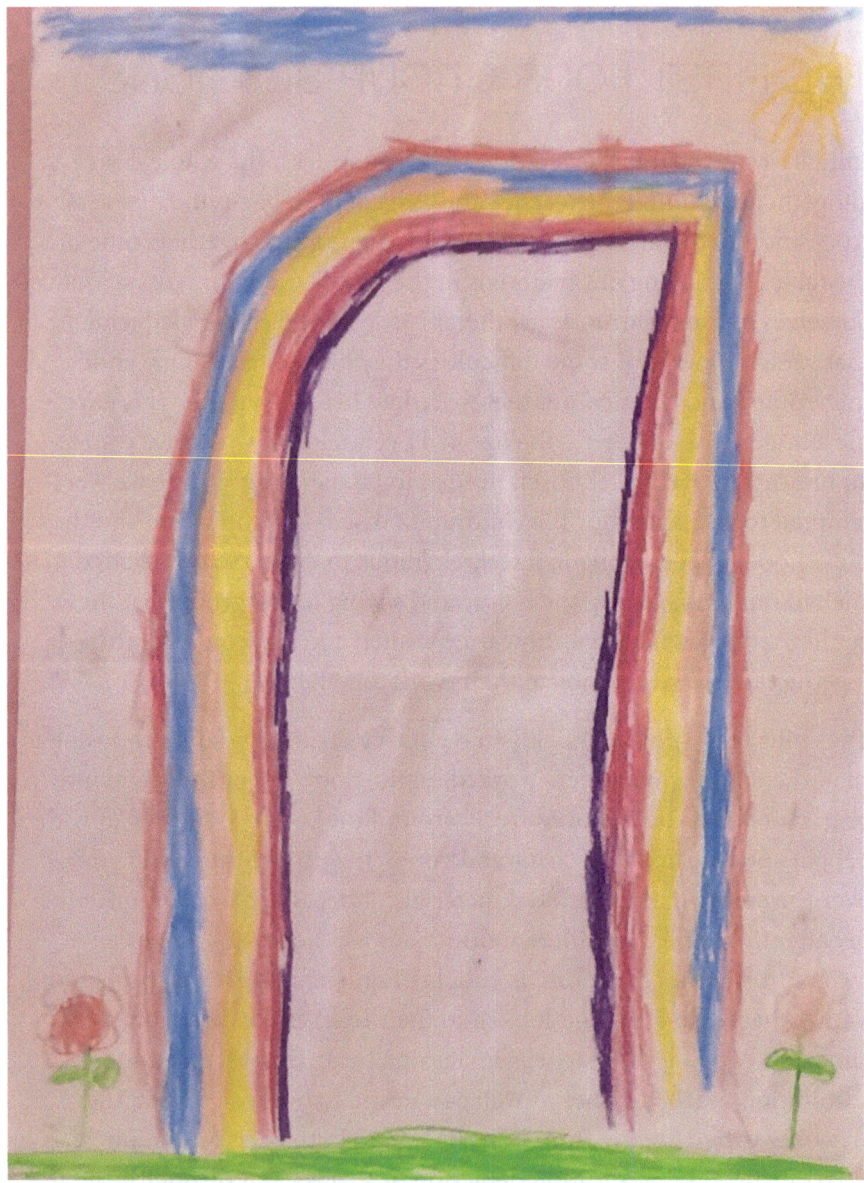

Figure 6.1 *Rainbow. Artwork made by a group member.*

We encouraged the class to come together for the end of the group to look at the art, but the children simultaneously competed with, and ignored, each other. When one child forcefully kicked another, the teacher took over the leadership, telling the children she was upset with their behaviour and warning them that my co-therapist and I would not want to come back if they continued to misbehave. I felt like a child who had come to play, with the parent threatening to end future playdates, a reflection of my anxiety about the future of the group.

While our view was that group anxieties could be contained through the provision of a space for the children to play out some of their rivalrous feelings, we worried that the management team would see the teacher's intervention as our having lost control of the class. As a result, we decided to split the class into two groups (groups A and B). In attempting to make the children's behaviour more manageable we were responding to the school's need for more order, but we were also, perhaps, responding to the children's need for more attention.

GROUP A AFTER HALF TERM

I will now focus on just Group A, which included the teaching assistant and was facilitated by my co-therapist and I. The sessions now took place in a building separate from the main school, which was new to the children and felt very different from their classroom. We grouped together tables for art making to form one large table in the middle of the room, but started and ended the group sitting together on large comfy sofas where we could place the artwork in the middle. A visual clue as to how young the children were was how small they were against the height of the tables and chairs in the room. Being faced with this and thoughts of their innocence and loss was very upsetting for me. I wondered whether my own hopes and expectations for the group were too high and whether this was an additional pressure for them to perform.

At the start of each session, we spent a short time discussing the boundaries of the group. One boundary was the request that the children try and remain in the room throughout. In the first session, one boy, pointing to the distinctive fire exit, said we shouldn't 'ever leave through that door as you would get lost'. The group became fixated with this door and it became a repeated narrative from the children week after week. Interestingly, the same happened in the other group. We understood this as a way for the children to let us know about some of their anxieties in relation to the fire, yet the specifics of what the door symbolised to them were unknown to us until a later session.

After the art making, it was always difficult for the group to come back together, with some children taking a considerable amount of time and needing to be called by the other group members. Listening to each other continued to be especially hard, and there was an ongoing rivalry for the adults' attention. I would often feel overwhelmed as my own voice could not be heard over the noise. The images continued to include creatures in remote fantastical habitats, as if thinking about the creatures together in previous sessions had opened up a larger and perilous landscape which was difficult to navigate. Maps were often made and then rolled up with the persistent request that they took them away with them. The groups left me exhausted. In tidying up the debris, Alice and I would often find tiny images on small pieces of paper that littered the floor. We collected these as important fragments of the group.

During session eight, Zain[1] became increasingly tearful. As the children around him drew dinosaurs, he pleaded with me to draw one for him as his own work wasn't pleasing enough. A powerful feeling that I was being cruel was evoked as I sat, resisting the urge to draw something, withholding what he pleaded for, as I attempted to stay focused on the group. Haris and Yousef tried to help Zain and it was wonderful to witness the children working together in an attempt to provide some resolution, but Zain remained unsatisfied.

Over time it seemed easier to come together and the children brought elaborate narratives to their images, which they started to enjoy thinking

---

1 Patient/institutional identities. Names, biographical details and other identifiers have been changed in respect to confidentiality.

about together. In session twelve, when Leila presented herself in her image trapped inside the stomach of a whale, the group were quick to provide suggestions as to how to get her out, demonstrating their increased ability to be with, and aid, each other's distress. Thinking back to the class we had observed in December, they seemed like a different group of children – there was a sense we were getting to know the children's experiences and they were beginning to be understood by both ourselves and their peers. This was also reflected by their teacher and TA who shared encouraging anecdotes of the children with us.

THE ANNIVERSARY OF THE FIRE

As the anniversary of the fire approached the weather grew warmer, a visceral reminder of the previous year. The surrounding area was being decorated with green hearts and emblems, which appeared to heighten the feeling of anxiety both in the group and within the school. Alice and I were asked to join a meeting with the management team who were trying to decide how best the school could observe the anniversary. The team seemed anxious to balance celebrating those they had lost whilst recognising the sorrow still present in the community. Again, they were worried about the impact this could have on the children, warning us they did not want to have the children in tears at the memorial. I wondered if we'd been invited to the meeting to witness the complexity of decisions they faced and to be sure we would hold them in mind through this uncertain and difficult time. During this meeting I believe it was the first time I had heard the management use the name of the child who had died in the fire. This felt extremely powerful to hear.

Session fifteen took place two days before the anniversary. Alice and I named this for the children at the start of the group, suggesting it might cause an arousal of different feelings. During the art making Khalid quietly showed me his image, which was of a lion woken in the night to a fire. I said, "Lions are usually strong and fierce, I wonder how this one is feeling?", he simply said, "I'm the lion". Later Khalid revealed to the group that he and his family had been evacuated during the night and had been living in a hotel ever since. In a troubled voice, Harris asked Khalid what had happened to all his toys. It was then the children shared their fantasies about how their friend had died in the fire. They thought she had died when trying to escape from the fire because the darkness and smoke had separated her from her family. Listening to their accounts was incredibly hard, some children cried while others admitted they were confused as they hadn't witnessed the fire itself. The significance of not leaving through the fire door became clear, and the map making seemed to symbolise a means of preventing children from becoming lost from the group. The children had been demonstrating ways to keep themselves safe when the outside world was so frightening.

As the summer holiday approached, Alice and I pressed the management team for a decision as to whether the group would end or continue in September. We proposed continuing the group to support the children's transition into the next academic year, given the difficulty they'd had settling into year one.

A meeting was arranged with the SENCo, the class teacher and a senior leader, who was also going to be the class teacher in year two. In preparation, we provided a detailed report illustrating the changes we'd seen in the class since we had begun the group. While discussing this the class teacher gave her support for art therapy and shared her insight into the class. The senior leader then became fixated on needing to know whether a particular image (Figure 6.2) was that of 'Grenfell Tower', asking, 'did they (the child) actually say it was?' In my response I explained it didn't really matter whether this was Grenfell Tower, that actually it could be any tower, as Grenfell will remain part of the children's life landscape. Despite this, even if the children had not witnessed the fire, seeing the tower above their school and being aware of what happened must be very frightening. These children live in similar blocks and towers – it was clear from the group that they worry if the same thing could happen again. The senior leader remained sceptical, and remained focused on the connection to the Grenfell Tower needing

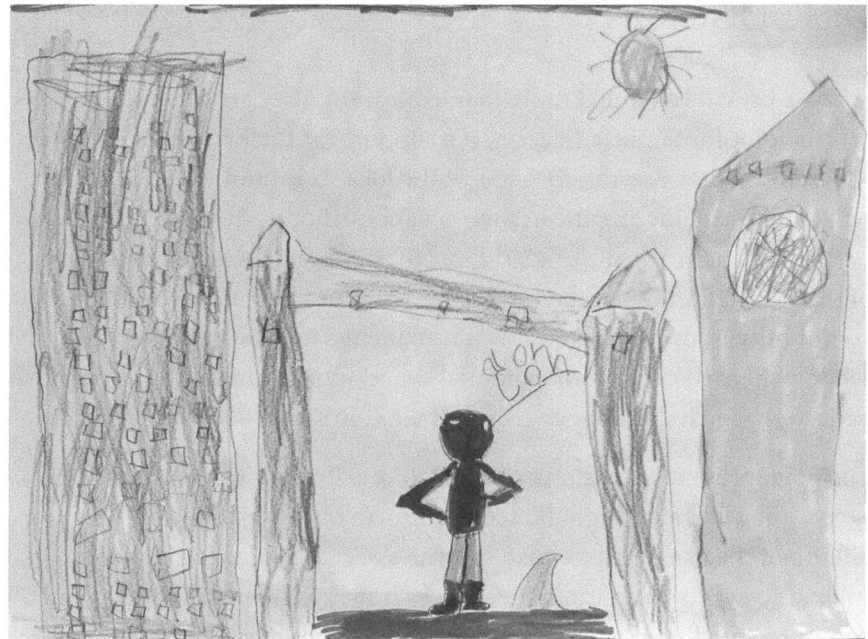

Figure 6.2 London. Artwork made by a group member.

to be explicit. Further requests for rational knowledge and objectivity were made, which could not be satisfied by our symbolic understandings nor by the changes of behaviour we described in the class. I worried that not only was my own professional voice not being heard, neither were the voices of the children.

Following the return to school in the new academic year we learned that the management had changed their decision and decided not to continue with the group after all. The senior leader told us that the children had moved on and as their new class teacher, she felt able to deal with the class. I felt the importance of the ending process, discussed in our meeting, was being denied, and so too was the relationship the children had established with my co-therapist and I. It felt appropriate to negotiate more time as we had informed the children we would be coming back. I'm thankful that six more sessions were therefore agreed in order to end the group.

DISCUSSION

Schools provide so much more than education; they are often the centre point for families in accessing support for further needs. As Rita Klein notes, they are 'microcosms of the local communities they serve, reflecting the demographic of their neighbourhoods in all their diversity, challenges and inequalities' (2012, p. 60). If the school is a microcosm of the local community, then our experience in this school reflects a community in deep conflict. It was a challenge to provide therapy within a school where the notion of 'potential space' was at odds with the prevalent pedagogy which denies the voice of their children.

The management request not to speak of the fire, while framed as protecting children, might be seen as a form of denial. Case (1987), talking of the use of euphemisms or the avoidance of talking of traumatic events to children, references Bowlby's research (1981), which demonstrated that if grief is not worked through in childhood there are inevitable repercussions in adult life. From the school's point of view, my co-therapist and I were there to bring a sense of unity to the children who were not getting along. Yet, for us, the children's unmanageable behaviour could only be understood as a response to the fire and avoidance of speaking about it would only exacerbate their distress.

For weeks I felt we were failing to meet the school's expectations as we could not get the children to sit and listen to each other, despite having split the class. I worried we were running out of time and the team would end the group. However, experiencing the group as out of control might have been the children's way of communicating what everyone was feeling, helpless, exemplified by Zain's desperation that I draw for him.

As indicated by the repeated map drawing, we felt the children were in desperate need for the adults to map a safe way out of their territory full of dinosaurs. It was significant that neither my co-therapist nor myself had been told in the referral that a child in the class had died or that there was a survivor of the fire in the group. That we had learnt this from the child himself, shows that the responsibility of naming traumatic events had been left to the children. As the sessions progressed the children appeared increasingly able to tolerate each other, coinciding with a growing sense that the trauma, a dangerous territory, could be mapped, named and collectively felt.

Trauma, distress and denial are not the only ways of understanding this experience. The ongoing complaints from the parents stayed with me. There seemed to be a parallel between their dissatisfaction with the school and the community's conflict with the council. Anger at the local authority was evident at public meetings, such as the Grenfell Recovery Scrutiny Committee, and on social media. The anguish in the community was clear as they waited for answers from officials, speculation grew as to how many people had lost their lives and what had caused the fire to spread so quickly. The children continually questioned whether the fire door would lead them to safety, which resounded with the community's feeling that the authorities had failed to keep them safe. The instruction to 'stay put' was now evidently so wrong it must have been deeply confusing for the children (and adults) to know who and what to trust.

The decision to end the group was explained as a need to prioritise the children's formal learning; the school risks punishment if it fails to conform to certain academic standards. The national curriculum has become increasingly restrictive, designed to measure what is taught, or rather designed to teach what can be measured. As children move up the education system, the space for play is eroded. The school's management would have felt a growing pressure for this class to get back to learning, in order not to risk being deemed a 'failing school'. The pressure to produce results leads to a state of hyper-rationality, where 'rule following comes to triumph over questioning and thinking' (Dalal, 2018, p. 3). In this heavily regulated system, we can see why play, imagination and symbols are met with scepticism, and with it, the voice of the children is left unheard.

Under UK law schools are expected to refrain from expressing political views, but considering the fire without the context in which it took place seemed impossible. The fire was an inherently political event and it may have felt dangerous to mention it at all. Alice and I may have represented something dangerous to the school. LCAT is an organisation born out of a disaster, perhaps seen as radical in comparison to other bureaucratic pathways on offer within the mental health system. LCAT is political as it prioritises the voices of the community it is part of. The work, through art, gave voice to the children, to express their fears and helplessness, and gave the opportunity to find ways to be with and help each other.

The fire caused great distress throughout the community, and management's requests of us should be seen in the context of disaster. It is important to remember that the staff in the school would likely have been in a state of trauma themselves, with the school being left with little additional support or resources to care for itself or for the children. For the school, attempting to regulate and regain control of the class should be seen as a way of coping with this extraordinary distress. How could we possibly provide any speedy resolution for the children or the school when so many injustices from the fire remained ongoing within the community?

In spite of these difficulties, LCAT continues to provide an art psychotherapy service to an increasing number of primary and secondary schools in North Kensington, including this one.

ACKNOWLEDGEMENT

I would like to express my heartfelt gratitude to Alice Patrick for her unquestionable support, thinking and co-facilitation of the group.

REFERENCES

Bowlby, J. (1981). *Attachment and Loss: Vol. 3. Loss: Sadness and Depression.* Harmondsworth: Penguin.

Case, C. (1987). A Seacrh for Meaning: Loss and Transition in Art Therapy with Children. In: Dalley, T., Case, C., Schaverien, J., Weir, F., Halliday, D., Hall, P.N. and Waller, D. (eds), *Images of Art Therapy: New Developments in Theory and Practice.* 1st ed., London: Tavistock Publications, pp. 36–73.

Dalal, F. (2018). *CBT: The Cognitive Behavioural Tsunami: Managerialism, Politics and the Corruptions of Science.* 1st ed., London and New York: Routledge.

Klein, R. (2012). *Therapeutic Practice in Schools.* 1st ed., London: Routledge.

Reddick, D. (2008). Working with the Whole Class in Primary Schools. In: Case, C. and Dalley, T. (eds), *Art Therapy with Children: From Infancy to Adolescence.* London: Routledge, pp. 86–102.

PART THREE

Against all odds

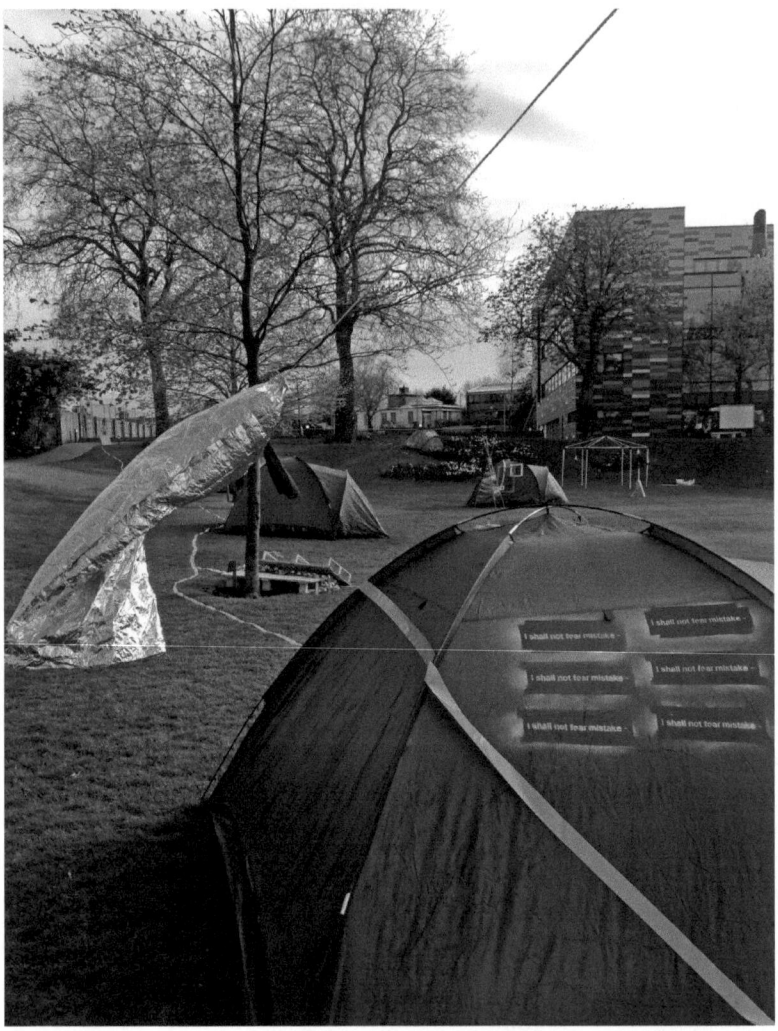

Figure P.3 *View of the Field: Goldsmiths University, April 2016. Photograph by Lesley Morris.*

'Crossing the field' was a participatory artwork made at the 2016 Art Therapy Conference: Finding Spaces, Making Places. The piece aimed to explore the cultural and political significance of the conference themes. Provoked by the global crisis of whole populations of people seeking safety and refuge and evocative of the 2011 Occupy protests, tents were used to home temporary and evolving exhibitions made spontaneously by conference delegates over the three-day conference.

CHAPTER SEVEN

A place of safety or a hostile environment?

How enactment in an art psychotherapy group revealed impacts of immigration controls on the mental health of asylum seekers and migrants detained in a psychiatric unit

Annamaria Cavaliero

DOI: 10.4324/9781003107408-10

INTRODUCTION

People who are seeking asylum because of persecution in their own countries and who experience mental illness very often find the bureaucracy they encounter in the UK contributes to their psychological disturbance. When an asylum seeker with no recourse to public funds is admitted to psychiatric hospital, this may be a culmination of many forms of stress on top of the trauma of having to flee their home country and the difficulties of the journey to asylum. This affects how they experience the help they are given. If accessing mental health support feels risky due to the suspicion that the National Health Service (NHS) will share data with the Home Office (HO), many prefer not to take that option and may become seriously ill before they encounter mental health services. The imposition of charges way beyond the capacity of a person's ability to pay is another serious deterrent to their seeking and receiving timely medical interventions (Campbell, 2020). Although asylum seekers are exempt from charges, failed asylum seekers are not.

Reynolds and Mitchell (2019) also highlight the corrosive moral implications of the National Health Service's enforcement of charges for medical care to 'overseas visitors'.

> Following the introduction of the data sharing MOU [Memorandum of Understanding] and with increasing securitisation of the health system via the charging regulations, faith in medical confidentiality has been disrupted. Patients are not seeking necessary healthcare such as antenatal care unless they reach crisis point or they may under-report symptoms, leading to worse health outcomes, presentation of more advanced disease and increased transmission of communicable diseases.
> (Reynolds and Mitchell, 2019, p. 500)

The imperatives of the HO regarding migrants and asylum seekers have also significantly impacted the professional integrity of health and legal professionals as a high degree of trust is needed in their relationships with their clients. Professionals have been left distressed and encumbered in their efforts to offer meaningful help to this vulnerable population.

In this chapter I consider how a ward-based group can be affected by the demands of other staff members. Ward staff have various jobs to do and sometimes find it hard to wait for patients to become free. Sometimes the group clashes with other necessary activities such as the ward round. While patients are usually keen to be seen in ward rounds, as they can find out about their treatment, leave and potential discharge, not every patient welcomes this. I describe how power dynamics, due to competing ward agendas, in an art therapy group revealed, in an embodied way, just how connected the hospital had become with the HO and border police in the minds of some patients. I will present a vignette from clinical practice that shows how the external political world can get enacted in therapy and how this impacts patients and therapists.

CONTEXT

The broader cultural setting of a hostile environment for migrants, either asylum seekers or economic migrants, has been in place, at least, since 2010, supposedly as a deterrent to illegal migration. The media's reportage using terms such as swarming, 'fleeing, sneaking, flooding' (Gabrielatos and Baker, 2008) has served as a means of 'othering' human beings who have come to this country seeking asylum from persecution or in an attempt to escape material poverty. It has been used as a political means to stigmatise migrants, through the use of language such as 'fraudulent' asylum claims, serving to delegitimise migrants and asylum seekers in much of the public sphere. This has been accompanied by a hardening of policy denying migrants and asylum seekers rights to housing, employment, legal aid, health care, education and benefits. An element of this hostile environment has been the de facto denial of Legal Aid to asylum seekers since 2012 (Grierson, 2018).

Even if a person has indefinite leave to remain, this can be revoked if there is a criminal offence. When a person is psychologically very unwell, they may be involved in some minor infringement of the law. The lack of legal services available now makes migrants and asylum seekers extremely vulnerable in criminal cases as their recourse to legal support is extremely limited. The Legal Aid, Sentencing and Punishment of Offenders Act in 2012 cut access to legal aid by making it difficult for solicitors to take on cases on a pro bono basis, disempowering asylum seekers and migrants even further.

Even seeking legal aid, housing and health care can be experienced as terrifying, as institutions including landlords, legal aid providers and, crucially, the NHS were obliged to carry out identity checks for the HO. This means that those people with irregular immigration status often fear encounters with authority and bureaucracy and distrust all institutions and authority figures, including the NHS and health professionals. Institutional bureaucracy has become a frontline of immigration control, meaning those seeking to access services are treated as objects of suspicion.

This not only poses ethical dilemmas for practitioners and institutions whose aim is to help those in need, but also very real consequences if they choose not to comply. It is also a real issue that asylum seekers face detention and deportation, and if they cannot trust those they need help from they will avoid seeking it. In 2018, under pressure from the human rights' NGO Liberty, the Home Office finally suspended the agreement requiring the NHS to pass on data belonging to migrants suspected of not having legal status. However, trust in the NHS remains seriously eroded (Usborne, 2018).

All asylum seekers and migrants face this increasingly hostile environment, but a group of this population may also develop serious mental health problems, which can involve disturbance to such an extent that they are admitted to psychiatric wards. While there are other contributory factors, the stress of being without funds and support, ineligible for legal aid, housing, education, employment or medical treatment, can create the perfect storm of circumstances leading to mental breakdown.

Research suggests that asylum seekers and refugees are more likely to experience poor mental health than the local population, including higher rates of depression, PTSD and other anxiety disorders. Increased vulnerability to mental health problems is linked to both pre-migration experiences, in particular exposure to war trauma, and the post-migration conditions that refugees often face, including separation from family, difficulties with asylum procedures or detention, unemployment and inadequate housing.

(Mental Health Foundation, 2016, p. 43)

While not all of these people are sectioned, one of the most traumatising ways that they may encounter mental health services is through section 136 of the Mental Health Act, which empowers the police to bring people into hospital. It is ironic in the case of asylum seekers suffering a mental health crisis that they are taken to what is called a 'place of safety'.

Their route into hospital may equally have been under a different kind of section or informally (voluntary). While less traumatic it will still involve a loss of liberty, which they may equate with other forms of bureaucracy they have previously encountered, for example detention. Therefore, how they experience the psychiatric unit may include different dimensions that affect their behaviour and attitude to professionals and other patients, adding another layer to their diagnosis and/or symptoms. These sets of procedures reinforce the sense of disempowerment and lack of agency that many asylum seeker patients may feel on encountering police, social services and psychiatric teams.

DELIVERING ART PSYCHOTHERAPY IN ACUTE SETTINGS

Where I work the art psychotherapy provision is generally in the form of open groups which take place on the wards. This means that therapist/ client alliances may not be established. Patients may use the session as much or as little as they feel able due to their levels of psychological distress or confusion. Because the population on the ward, and thus in the group, varies from week to week, each session might function as a stand-alone event, and as such, carries great significance. The presence of severe psychopathology means that communication is often indirect and concrete; I need to be aware of the hostile internal structures at play and endeavour to minimise any responses that may mirror this externally. As a therapist I need to be aware of my own power status and position as a representative of the system in which patients find themselves.

In the case of asylum seeker patients, the external environment is already very uncertain, threatening and stressful; and in an acute state of psychosis the internal world may be equally terrifying and even less comprehensible. This adds further complication to the experience of the patient, as their perception is often extremely disturbed. On the wards, staff have operated within a medical and behavioural model, perhaps replicating a position of authority that asylum seekers and migrants have come to mistrust. As an art psychotherapist I offer an open and non-directive space. In the eyes of migrants and asylum seekers, of course, I may be seen as a person of authority who will do nothing to alleviate their situation and is only part of the hostile environment. An important element of my work is a willingness to understand this and tolerate projections onto me as a persecutory object. Often it is only by my accepting this that the patient can begin to work through their feelings of distrust and abandonment.

A SINGLE WARD-BASED ART THERAPY GROUP (2010)

The following vignette explores how an unwitting bureaucratic intervention recreated elements of trauma, such as distrust and fear, leading to flight, which re-enacted the hostile environment. This inadvertently contributed to a positive therapeutic alliance as the therapist was seen to be distant from the bureaucracy. All names have been removed to protect clients' identity, other identifying features have been disguised or fictionalised.

This was a group that I wrote up in detail afterwards as it had made me think a lot about the idea of the art room as container (Killick, 2000) and I was questioning how solid that container can be on an acute ward with the myriad agendas that battle for attention in the working day. It seems that interruptions are an on-going feature of the work in this setting, head counts and shop-run requests all threaten the sanctity of the therapy group. I have used door signs with many different ways of requesting privacy, explained the reasons for this to ward teams in person and by email, but in spite of this, I am often required to physically defend the privacy of the group. However, because of the particular circumstances of the patients who were accessing the art therapy group that day, and in light of the (then recent) imposition of the hostile environment, what happened in this group made me think about how invasions of a so-called safe space can have sinister connotations.

The open group on that day was well attended from the start of the session. I am a female white British art psychotherapist. The four group members included an Eastern European man (Mr O); a Central African man (Mr S); a South African man (Mr K); and a woman of Asian descent (Ms R).

Mr O was under the delusion that he had been mistakenly brought to hospital because another person had stolen his identity and left him with theirs. He was very mistrustful of staff but enjoyed art and had been attending the art therapy group for three weeks. Mr S had been isolative for weeks, believing that his life was in danger, but had recently started to engage with staff and patients. It was his first time in the group. Mr K had recently returned to hospital after relapsing in the community. At this time he was displaying some defensively manic behaviour. He had attended the group before. Ms R had been regularly attending art therapy sessions for about two months; she had originally been very unwell and also mistrustful of the white therapist but had now established a greater sense of trust and made great improvements in her mental state.

The group members engaged quickly with the art materials except Mr O, who spent some time looking at a magazine. The atmosphere in the room was calm and engaged.

Ms R, who was waiting to be rehoused, was making an image of a row of houses with curtains in the windows and leafy trees outside. This was in contrast to her earlier images, which were very chaotic, incorporating many words and fractured imagery.

Mr S was drawing a row of stick people with red dots in their chest area and he identified the central figure as himself. He drew a red circle in the central area of this figure too. He showed me his image, saying the row of people were his friends. I asked him what the red dot signified and he said it was his stomach. Then he drew another figure underneath and wrote '6000+' next to it. He handed me his image. I asked him what the number related to. When he did not reply I wondered whether it might be the number of people from the persecuted group in his country who were, at that time, seeking asylum in the UK. Mr S did not answer but scribbled over the central figure with black crayon as if to hide it. He then added a figure of a woman in pink crayon, and said this woman was a big problem for him.

Mr K was a little elated and finding it hard to settle, he was talking a lot and had at one point stated, 'Don't lose your job, if you lose your job you lose your family, if you lose your family you will become homeless.' I commented that it sounded like a cycle. He said that he would break the cycle and started to make a circular image, as if to depict this cycle. Mr O was not joining in the conversations.

At this point in the group a male nurse opened the door without knocking and leaned into the space and called Mr O to come out of the session to join the ward round. Mr O refused and became quickly aroused. He started to speak loudly to the nurse. I went to the door and asked the nurse if he could call him after the session had finished. The nurse then left but returned a few minutes later with a doctor and an entourage of men and women, most likely his students. Standing outside the door to the room he tried to get Mr O to leave the session, again interrupting the session. Mr O was adamant that he would not go and shouted that they should contact the police to clear up the case of mistaken identity. At this point the other group members became highly nervous and aroused and all started to leave the session through the door with the doctor and his entourage on the other side still trying to get Mr O to come out. I expressed my frustration that the group had now disintegrated and explained to the doctor that this can be what happens when a therapy session is interrupted. The containing space is no longer able to function as such and people start to feel unsafe. He apologised and seemed genuinely regretful but explained that he had been trying to see this man for nearly a year. The only person left in the room was Mr O; I said that I would try to talk to him in the session. The doctor also expressed surprise that the group should be 'so fragile' and apologised for disrupting it.

When I spoke to Mr O he told me that if I tried to get him to speak to the doctors he would no longer be able to trust me, and that this would mean he would no longer 'be able to come to the group'. I acknowledged that the group should not have been interrupted and apologised. After a while it became evident that Mr O was not going to leave the session and the doctor and his entourage left the vicinity of the room.

After this I was very relieved to find that all the group members returned to the group and continued to work on their images. Mr O, who had not been painting when the group was interrupted, started to cover a sheet of paper with gold paint, using a brush, seemingly to express some of his pent-up feeling. Mr S came back and took the silver paint and started to cover a sheet of paper as well. Ms R added some words to her picture expressing some rather paranoid thoughts; she had been doing this all over her imagery when she was especially unwell but had recently started to make purely pictorial images. At this point the group started to talk about 'illegal immigrants'. Mr O said that he was being treated like an illegal immigrant. Both Mr S and Mr K were anxious about their status in this country. Mr K said, 'We are not illegal immigrants we are people.'

I ended the group by acknowledging the effect that the interruption had on the group and expressing pleasure that it had regrouped and continued despite this.

After the session I spoke to the ward round staff about how the interruption had affected the group. I said that I hoped that we could work together in future to prevent such a thing happening again. Mr O himself had put into words exactly what he wanted from the group – and I felt that he was speaking for the other group members too, although most likely that was not his intention – when he said he wanted to come to a place where he could start to allow himself to trust people. I expressed my sense of upset that group members had been exposed to a situation that could evoke real terror in the light of their experience as migrants and asylum seekers in this country.

REFLECTION

I was curious as to who the pink woman in Mr S's drawing might be and wondered if it might be me – the therapist going too quickly to interpret the imagery. My other thought was that it might represent the Home Secretary who had recently introduced the term 'hostile environment' with regard to illegal immigrants. Whatever the case, I was aware of my position as white British female therapist in the group and what this might represent. It was interesting how, when the group re-formed, the actual term illegal immigrant entered the conversation. Mr O introduced it; I felt he was trying to differentiate himself from his co-participants, implying that he was a legal migrant whereas Mr S and Mr K, and even possibly Ms R, in his mind, may have been illegal. Mr K brought in the sense of the group's shared humanity by saying 'we are not illegal immigrants, we are people.'

I felt that the function of the group as a place where thoughts and feelings could be communicated, thought about and digested by the therapist and group had been temporarily ruptured by the interruption. It had survived the first intrusion by the nurse but when the doctor arrived at the door with his entourage, the room started to feel very dangerous. My refusal to admit entry to these professionals may have modelled that the space was being defended but it still became too claustrophobic for the group participants to endure. They needed to escape. That there was a group of people at the exit added to the sense of danger and fear. It took this enactment of a terrorised group for the doctor to understand the effect of the interruption. Although this was clearly not his intention, I don't think it is an exaggeration to say that the interruption was experienced as a raid on the group. I wondered why there had been surprise at the fact that the group was fragile. Perhaps there is a lack of appreciation of how, in art psychotherapy, participants can become very deeply involved in their own material and a disturbance from outside can be extremely jarring. When the group is made up of people who have a sense of their own vulnerability to authority and are hyper vigilant, this can actually be terrifying. It may also be that this out of character lack of awareness was created by the pressures of the hostile environment on this team. David Bell describes the government as an 'ever present ... hovering ... menacing superego penetrating into every pore of the relationships within the system' (2013, p. 251). It is a fact that the government has very real powers over how the NHS functions.

In my previous work as an art psychotherapist co-facilitating an art therapy group for women survivors of torture and political violence, group members told us about the lack of privacy in the accommodation they lived in while awaiting a decision on their asylum claims. They never knew when the landlords might enter their home. For some this echoed the experience of being held in detention on arrival in this country when staff were able to enter their rooms without knocking at any time of the day and night. The terror that this evoked was intense in case it meant they were to be forcibly deported. It may also have replicated something of their experiences before leaving their countries of origin, when danger to life was extremely real. I thought about how, in his mental distress, Mr S was afraid that people wanted to kill him. Just when he was expressing something in his art about being an asylum seeker, the door was opened by a member of the nursing staff, shortly followed by a doctor and a group of besuited people. I thought about the possible conflation in his mind of these staff with governmental authority figures who had critical powers over his future. In his image, Mr S had drawn people with red dots on their bodies – I thought these red dots looked like the sights of a sniper's rifle. He was very afraid that people wanted to kill him. And with the threat of deportation being real, this could not only be understood as paranoid delusion.

Ms R had been very unwell when she was sectioned under the Mental Health Act and detained in the hospital. Her illness had manifested itself in such paranoid delusions that she had felt the need to defend herself and her home in a concrete way, covering the doors and windows with homemade placards and wearing many layers of clothing and attached items. Some of her paranoia was to do with different countries representing possibly dangerous powers in the world, and some were of her own person being invaded and spied upon at all moments. For a while she was very mistrustful of the therapist, but her need to express herself using the art materials was strong and, perhaps because I allowed and considered her powerful projections, the room became tolerable for her to be in. She had reached the point where these projections had lost their potency and she was able to regard me in a much less distrustful way when the interruption occurred. It was striking that she was making an image of a row of terraced houses at the time. I doubted that she would have been able to return to the group after the doctor and his entourage left had she not worked through her feelings about the therapist over time. The fact that she started to write words of a paranoid nature over her imagery indicated that her newly established sense of safety in the room had been disturbed.

Mr K had been in this country for work when he had a breakdown and was sectioned under the Mental Health Act in hospital. Becoming seriously unwell while on a work visa meant that his legal status was uncertain, as was his status as provider for his family. On his second admission, he was beginning to use the group to face some difficult realities that his illness had been defending him from up until then. It felt as if the interruption had ambushed this important moment. Luckily it had not derailed the group completely.

The use by two group members of gold and silver paint applied in long brushstrokes and covering the full sheets of paper seemed to serve some kind of self-soothing purpose for the individuals; that it happened after the group had reformed may also symbolise something precious that was not destroyed.

Reflecting on how the ward environment, with its lack of respect for the boundaries of psychotherapy groups, might actually re-traumatise vulnerable patients leads me to conclude that there is room for learning here.

CONCLUSION

The pressure on art psychotherapists to deliver sessions on many wards means that they are not always able to attend ward team meetings, but feeding back after sessions is important. In the above case I felt it was necessary to respond to the senior clinicians who had not accepted the patient's choice not to attend ward round, to show how this action had resulted in the fragmentation of the group. The competing agenda was the need for this doctor to meet his institutional demands, but it felt as if he had taken advantage of the patient having left his room to attend a therapy group and that the repeated interruption of this space was seen as acceptable. That it happened at a time when the NHS was being pressured by government imperatives may also have played a part in this. Art psychotherapists are well placed to get a more holistic view of a patient and what is disturbing them, and this should be fed back to teams. As Evans recommends, 'Clinical staff teams need time to reflect on their practice in shift handover and ward rounds' (2016, p. 84). Art psychotherapists ideally would contribute to this process and where I work there have been some positive moves in this direction, with art psychotherapists now contributing to case formulations. However, the frequency of staff turnover means this is an ongoing and, at times, demoralising effort. I mentioned that art therapists have a less medically defined role that can make it helpful for engaging with patients, but it can also mean that staff don't always understand our clinical requirements and the contributions to team thinking that art therapy offers.

Art psychotherapists on inpatient wards need to be prepared to accept that they may be seen as part of the bureaucracy that has negatively affected the wellbeing and safety of the asylum seeker. They also need to defend the group against interruption from competing agendas on the wards. Advocating for the mental health of patients is a vital element of our role. Something which is gaining currency in my workplace in terms of attitudes towards mental health treatment is the concept of 'trauma-informed treatment'. All staff are encouraged to promote this in their interactions with patients.

> The current mental health system tends to conceptualise extreme behaviours and distress as symptoms of mental illnesses, rather than as coping adaptations to past or current traumas. As a consequence, responses to people in extreme distress can be unhelpful and even (re)traumatising ... less obvious forms of (re)traumatising include the use of 'power-over' relationships that replicate power and powerlessness by disregarding the experience, views and preferences of the individual.
>
> (Sweeney et al., 2018, p. 332)

The system in which we work may make us all complicit in the enactment and enforcement of the hostile environment. While resisting governmental and institutional imperatives does not always feel safe for professionals and clinicians, through our training, supervision and continued professional development, art psychotherapists working in this field should sustain awareness of the complex power dynamics at play for asylum seekers and migrants in the context of mental health services. Underpinning this is acknowledging that we work within an environment that can often feel hostile to service providers as well as service users.

REFERENCES

Bell, D. (2013). The Dynamics of Containment. In: Bell, D. and Novakovic, A. (eds), *Living on the Border: Psychotic Processes in the Individual, the Couple and the Group.* London: The Tavistock Clinic Series, Karnac, pp. 226–242.

Campbell, D. (2020). Migrants in the UK denied NHS care for average of 37 weeks, research finds. *The Guardian*, 14th October [online]. Available at: https://www.theguardian.com/society/2020/oct/14/migrants-denied-nhs-care-for-average-of-37-weeks-research-finds?CMP=Share_iOSApp_Other [Accessed 14 October 2020].

Evans, M. (2016). *Making Room for Madness in Mental Health: The Psychoanalytic Understanding of Psychotic Communication*. London: Karnac Books.

Gabrielatos, C. and Baker, P. (2008). Fleeing, sneaking, flooding: A corpus analysis of discursive constructions of refugees and asylum seekers in the UK press, 1996–2005. *Journal of English Linguistics*, 36(1), pp. 5–38.

Grierson, J. (2018). Lack of legal aid puts asylum seekers' lives at risk, charity warns. *The Guardian*, 19th July [online]. Available at: https://www.theguardian.com/law/2018/jul/19/lack-legal-aid-puts-asylum-seekers-lives-at-risk-charity-warns [Accessed 19 July 2018].

Killick, K. (2000). The Art Room as Container in Analytic Art Psychotherapy. In: Gilroy, A. and McNeilly, G. (eds), *The Changing Shape of Art Therapy*. London: Jessica Kingsley Publishers, pp. 99–114.

Mental Health Foundation (2016). Fundamental Facts About Mental Health 2016. Mental Health Foundation: London. Available at: https://www.mentalhealth.org.uk/publications/fundamental-facts-about-mental-health-2016 [Accessed 20 November 2018].

Reynolds, J.M.K. and Mitchell, C. (2019). 'Inglan is a bitch': Hostile NHS charging regulations contravene the ethical principles of the medical profession. *Journal of Medical Ethics*, 45, pp. 497–503. Available at: https://jme.bmj.com/content/45/8/497.full [Accessed 7 January 2021].

Sweeney, A., Filson, B., Kennedy, A., Collinson, L. and Gillard, S. (2018). A paradigm shift: Relationships in trauma-informed mental health services. *BJPsych Advances*, 24, pp. 319–333.

Usborne. C. (2018). 'How the hostile environment crept into schools, hospitals and homes'. *The Guardian*, 1st August. Available at: https://www.theguardian.com/uk-news/2018/aug/01/hostile-environment-immigrants-crept-into-schools-hospitals-homes-border-guards [Accessed 1st August 2018].

CHAPTER EIGHT

Prison cells
Transgenerational trauma and art psychotherapy groups with women in prison

Jessica Collier

DOI: 10.4324/9781003107408-11

'My mother groan'd! my father wept.
Into the dangerous world I leapt ...'

William Blake, 'Infant Sorrow', from *Songs*
of Innocence and of Experience (1794)

INTRODUCTION

For the majority of women in prison, distressing transgenerational experiences, characterised by physical and psychological deprivation, form the basis of their lived experience. Their trajectory in life is influenced by hostile political policies that augment their disadvantage and the impact of often traumatic and violent histories that may be passed down emotionally and epigenetically from their forebears. This hostile start in life, marked from conception by poverty, addiction, fragile mental health and societal prejudice, may lead to experiences in adulthood that amplify and repeat early disturbance and culminate in confinement to the institutionally hostile environment of prison. Here, women are removed from a society which itself is hostile to transgressions of perceived and accepted codes of femininity. In prison, the repeated abuse of power and trauma that led the women to be incarcerated in the first place may be unconsciously re-enacted by the institution itself and explored in art psychotherapy (Collier, 2015). Many women who spend time as adults incarcerated in prison cells may be born into a society that literally passes down prison 'cells'; the highest corollary for imprisonment being the imprisonment of a parent (Williams et al., 2012). The following chapter will elucidate this idea through a brief history of prison and society, a discussion of institutional disturbance, and vignettes of art psychotherapy groups failing and succeeding in a women's prison, highlighting how aggressive and hostile political and social policies impact on the pattern and escalation of external, material deprivation, as well as internal, emotional poverty.

THE PRISON ENVIRONMENT – AN HISTORICAL FOCUS

The history of modern prisons in the United Kingdom can be traced back to the eighteenth century. The Penitentiary Act of 1779 proposed incarceration in a state-run prison as an alternative to transportation to the penal colonies or the death sentence. So harsh was the treatment of criminals prior to this that progressive politicians voiced concerns 'that the unjust executions against the poor only served to increase their resentment against the richer classes' (Soothill, 2007, p. 34). Then, as now, it was the poor, the vulnerable and the oppressed who bore the brunt of society's inequality. Foucault delineated this pathway from physical torture to the taking of an individual's liberty, tracing the invention of the modern soul as a vehicle for sociological and philosophical concepts of retribution, from torture, to punishment and discipline, and finally to prison. The soul, suggests Foucault, 'is not born in sin and subject to punishment, but is born rather out of methods of punishment, supervision, and constraint' (Foucault, 1979, p. 29).

The intention, instrumentality and politics of imprisonment has gone around in circles throughout this time, depending on successive social mores and moral ideals. In the 1920s, reform and rehabilitation, and the idea that criminals should be treated well to support them to lead productive lives, became fashionable. Nevertheless, despite these humanitarian values, the reality was very different. The psychological deprivations and abuses and the decaying physical conditions led to riots, protests and escapes, and eventually resulted in the Woolf Report (1991), which insisted that 'a "just" prison could not be a place that makes offenders worse, but, rather, one that encourages self-respect and a sense of personal responsibility' (Scott, 2007, p. 58). This summons to treat prisoners humanely was, however, promptly undermined by the Conservative Prime Minister John Major, who declared that 'Society needs to condemn a little more and understand a little less' (Macintyre, 2011). This heralded a more austere and punitive approach. Secure custody once again became the primary aim of imprisonment; the consideration of social justice, human rights and alternative ways of responding to lawlessness as a consequence of poverty and oppression were diminished, and the most marginalised in society paid the price. 'Prisons in England and Wales disproportionately hold young people, property offenders, the mentally ill. Those who are unemployed or on benefits, those who are homeless or have been in care, and/or people disproportionately from black and minority ethnic communities' (cited in Scott, 2007, p. 68). In this list we must also include women who have been victims of violence and abuse, women living in poverty and women struggling with addictions.

AN INTERSECTIONAL FOCUS

When those who are incarcerated already experience suffering and hardship in society, as a result of explicit, implicit or systemic sexism, racism, misogyny, homophobia, disability or transphobia, and many other disadvantages including class and poverty, the punishment becomes exponentially more severe. Kimberle Crenshaw first used the term intersectionality in her influential paper 'Demarginalizing the intersection of race and sex: A Black feminist critique of antidiscrimination doctrine, feminist theory and antiracist politics' (1989), in which she suggested the metaphor of a crossroads to examine race and gender discrimination combined. This idea had been argued over many years by Black feminists, who noted that the specific experiences of Black women were excluded from feminist discourse. Since then, intersectionality has become a mainstream theory and one which may be helpful in understanding the severity of the hostile environment women experience in prison; 'incarceration or punishment comprises multiple intersections – not just of identity and power but of systemic dynamics that themselves do the work of subordination ... these systems work in tandem to create and justify conditions that render women vulnerable and subsequently punish them for their vulnerability' (Crenshaw, 2013, p. 25). Female offenders are treated differently to men. They are punished for transgressing their stereotypically compliant 'female' role in society and as such are deemed degenerate or immoral, frequently labelled as monstrous or depraved. This identity may be internalised by the women, manifesting in the harmful introjection of societal prejudices and revealed in critical and self-loathing imagery created during art psychotherapy (Collier, 2019b). Women from ethnic minorities face additional prejudice within the criminal justice system, being far more likely to be given a custodial sentence and having to serve longer than their White peers (Cox and Sacks-Jones, 2017). The historic subjugation of people of colour is linked to British colonialism and slavery. The unfounded structural fear of violence, the racist notion that Black women are 'strong' or 'crazy' (Maynard, 2018) and the moral castigation metered out to minority women by the judiciary could be seen as an introjection, on a systemic level, of the centuries of violence the White majority have committed upon them, and the unconscious terror of retaliation. In addition, women who have 'failed' to conform to stereotypical ideas of femininity are treated more harshly by the courts than women who exemplify their female role; 'conformity, both sexual and domestic, will invoke the court's benevolence, and it is this power to dispose, according to standards of normal female subjectivity in a patriarchal society, which characterises the discipline and punishment of women' (Medlicott, 2007, p. 253). Ultimately, this double-bind punishes women for being too 'feminine' or not 'feminine' enough (Smart, 1976). Undertaking art psychotherapy groups with these marginalised women in such a deeply hostile environment poses many challenges.

A WOMAN'S PLACE

'Women in prison are the recipients of contradictory and ideological control, based on familial, societal and masculinist assumptions' (Medlicott, 2007, p. 246). This reflects the way in which women are objectified in the general population and implies the complexity of what is or is not a hostile environment. For example, while women are considered to be risk averse, this is routinely measured from a white male perspective in a world where they have little to fear. For many women, every day may be fraught with risk depending on a number of factors, 'women routinely take risks … Going on a date can end in sexual assault. Leaving a marriage is financially, socially, and emotionally risky … being pregnant is about twenty times more likely to result in death than is a skydive' (Fine, 2018, p. 116). The issue here is to what extent women face a hostile environment at all times and the supposition that being held in prison is worse than having to survive in the community. On release, women have far worse outcomes than men, facing social exclusion and obstacles to employment, and hindered by lack of support due to the low numbers incarcerated and the consequent lack of investment (Carlen, 2012).

THE CYCLE OF CRIMINALITY AND DEPRIVATION

An estimated 17,000 children every year are put in care due to their mother being incarcerated (Prison Reform Trust, 2018). Their education may be disrupted, they may be separated from siblings, feel guilt, grief and shame, they may be abused and discriminated against. This intergenerational pattern is common in prison. It is an inescapable and normalised way of life. Given the hostility they face in the community, incarceration may seem the safer option as the majority of women in prison are survivors of gendered violence, physical or emotional abuse during childhood, and suffer from mental ill health and addiction (Women in Prison, n.d.). Of course, these traumatic histories do not justify the use of violence, the breaking of laws or the creation of further victims through offending. But for women given so little value in society, prison becomes their home; the staff and peers become their families; and their lives become a cycle of re-enactment.

CLINICAL WORK IN A HOSTILE ENVIRONMENT

AMBIVALENCE AND UNCONSCIOUS ATTACKS

Prisons are paradoxical institutions, where ambivalence and uncertainty are pervasive. To survive, women must internalise an identity which does not allow for vulnerability and the sharing of painful histories, especially in a group setting where their façade might be exposed or their experiences used against them. This makes the dynamic administration of art psychotherapy groups in prison particularly complex. Any prisoners who pose a danger to one another must be identified, and motivation to attend the group must be fully explored and understood. Trading and bullying are common, and maintaining a front of invulnerability is often considered more important than the prospect of improved mental health. In addition, prisoners are transferred unexpectedly, re-enacting losses and sudden endings in the therapy that may trigger responses that repeat earlier attachment traumas. When groups do get underway, they may face explicit hostility or opposition from the institution, or implicit attacks within the group itself. The former may manifest in rooms being made unavailable, staff entering spaces during therapy, officers refusing to unlock prisoners for sessions and so on. The prisoner's internal distress may be expelled by projecting it externally onto others (Klein, 1946), resulting in staff behaving harshly, 'even callously, as if in unthinking retaliation to the sense of being undermined or threatened' (Ruszczynski, 2012, p. 203). Unconscious envious attacks on the therapy space by overworked, traumatised staff, who may feel their own emotional needs are neglected, are a defensive response to the disturbing and unbearable projections they may receive on a daily basis; unacknowledged, unprocessed and leading to a highly toxic environment. Prison officers have wondered aloud to me why they don't get time, space and art materials. This was to such an extent that I once set up a regular studio group for security staff; a concrete reaction I hoped would mitigate the hostility. I sat for three months alone in the space, despite having advertised widely and handing out flyers on all the landings. By the fourth month, alone again, I went to see where the officers were, and found the custodial manager ripping up the flyers and putting them in the bin. The struggle to accept care is as strong in anxious and traumatised staff as it is in the women; one of many parallel processes taking place in prison. The paradox is that resisting emotional exposure as a survival strategy creates a less safe space, relationally and psychically; 'relational security is … about a readiness to join and actively participate in reflective interpersonal, and inter-professional, conversations within a wider culture of enquiry' (Scanlon, 2012, p. 224).

OPEN GROUP

When I started working in prison I 'inherited' an open group that had run for some time on the substance misuse landing. This was a high dependency unit accommodating newly incarcerated women withdrawing from alcohol and drugs, who were frequently ill, intoxicated, malnourished and confused. The physical location was the lowest point of the prison, in the semi-basement of the building; a long, dark corridor permeated with the strong odour of vomit, faeces and unwashed bodies. Each week the group was formed by the first eight women arriving in the room. This was extremely difficult to manage and contain. The art materials were stolen and drug dealing and medication trading was overt. The group was characterised by mess, chaos, loss and conflict. I began to dread the weekly set up. Intellectually, I was able to acknowledge that this feeling of dread, the disorder and degradation, might be a mirroring of the women's experience; a parallel process amplifying the waste and disorder of their lives. Emotionally, I felt exhausted and exploited; symptomatic perhaps of a deeply destructive projection that depleted my will to continue, as well as a concrete response to tiring and difficult work. I have found the psychoanalytic concept of projection, and particularly my understanding of projective identification (Klein, 1946), invaluable in helping mitigate the most profound and destructive feelings I experience in relation to my work with female offenders. For example, when working with women who have used violence, understanding the feelings of fear I might have in a session can serve as both an important way to assess risk in the moment and as a means to better understand that the women may fear the violent and destructive parts of themselves. If I were to consider my fear solely as my own reaction to material the women bring, or the environment in which I work, without considering my introjection of their frightening internal worlds, I might fail to appreciate how profoundly disturbing the intimacy and exposure of therapy might be for them. In addition, I might not consider my own projection of disturbing or unwanted parts of myself onto others.

A representative membership of the open group might include an HIV positive intravenous heroin user with leg ulceration; a young woman already afflicted with debilitating Korsakoff syndrome due to alcohol dependence; a malnourished sex worker beaten deaf by her pimp; numerous women who had lost their children; and, on one occasion, a homeless woman who I had once bought a cup of tea. She had sold her trainers for drugs. She didn't recognise me. This list does not aim to judge or caricature the women, but rather it exemplifies the physical and societal burdens they carried. Additionally, almost without exception, they had mental health diagnoses, most commonly personality disorder and post-traumatic stress disorder, habitually originating in childhood sexual abuse and transgenerational deprivation.

Typically, the women in the group would feel excited about using the materials and would often want to make a greeting card for the child they might have 'letterbox' contact with. During the ninety minutes, they would then become preoccupied with creating something for their often violent and abusive partner; taking great care and writing a loving message in their best handwriting. With ten minutes to go, they would realise they had neglected their child's birthday card and hurriedly, carelessly, throw together whatever happened to be left on the table, creating a botched mess and consequently feeling guilty and angry with themselves and with me. This happened so frequently that I came to see it as an unconscious re-enactment of their own childhood neglect and inability to prioritise those giving or needing care over those metering out abuse. Indeed, in individual art psychotherapy sessions, when they become aware that the childhood abusers they loved were actually harming them, and that this dynamic is being repeated in the institution, prisoners have frequently responded by accusing me of abusing or harming them, so unbearable is the emotional pain of this realisation (Collier, 2019a). In the open group, the time and consistency needed to work through this depth of betrayal was not available. The single session structure, sometimes utilised in open groups to conceive of and contain therapeutic factors such as hope, altruism, cohesiveness and catharsis (Yalom, 1975), did not seem possible to foster. So intense was the disturbance on this landing, so toxic were the projections from prisoners and staff, so impossible to contain was the anguish, that after a couple of years the psychic assaults and concrete reality became intolerable and I stopped running the sessions. I had learned that I could not contain a group with this level of unprocessed disturbance and lack of boundaries on my own, and with such limited support from the institution, and reflected that I may have unknowingly presided over, and perhaps colluded with, an unconscious re-enactment of chaotic, dysfunctional familial trauma and disturbance.

CLOSED PSYCHODYNAMIC GROUP AND THE 'ANTI-GROUP'

Not wanting to further enact this pattern of loss and neglect with the women, I established a closed group on the drug treatment landing, thus accommodating the same prisoners but further into their sentence and with a more stable membership. Titrating on methadone maintenance or detoxed from alcohol, the women were less volatile and the landing less chaotic. Nevertheless, while some of the women seemed more able to engage on an individual level, the system they were held within continued to work against the possibility of a functioning group.

Nitsun conceived the 'anti-group' (1991) partly in response to what he saw as group analysis founder S.H. Foulkes' unqualified optimism (Foulkes, 1948). Simply summarised, while Nitsun admired the group analytic emphasis on the importance of external and social, as well as internal factors, he felt there was not enough attention paid to the aggressive and destructive tendencies in societies, and hence in groups. Foulkes assumed that constructive forces in the group would direct it 'towards the norms of the community of which it is part' (Ibid, 1991, p. 9). However, the prison community cannot be perceived as 'normal'. Arguably, a society in which people continue to be locked up at great economic expense in dehumanising conditions might not be considered 'normal', though we can understand why this system endures – as Foucault's exploration of societal power and domination makes clear (1979) – and why it is particularly damaging for the female prison population, as described in Stewart and Collier's work documenting the lives of women in prison as told in the psychotherapy room (2019). The work of an analytic group is, in part, to transform the 'anti-group' by acknowledging and addressing the problems that may manifest frequently through complaints. 'Often this takes the form of attacks on the group; it is not good enough; it is second best ... it is directionless; there is no guidance; the presence of others with problems is a liability rather than an asset; it is an artificial situation; it gives too little time to the individual; it feels unsafe' (Nitsun, 1991, p. 12). Any art psychotherapist who has run groups will recognise these grievances and will have seen them worked through in a slow and sometimes painful process. These 'anti-group' dynamics may be particularly prevalent where the group members are locked up, making them 'temporarily excluded from the wider social group' (Sarra,1998, p. 85). However, in addition to this, with the members of the group living together in the same toxic environment, on the same landing and frequently in the same cell, the psychological exposure proved too much. The danger and disregard they felt was not a group process to be worked through but a concrete reality to be feared. Their emotional fragility and vulnerability, protected under their prison facades, was too raw to reveal. Brought up in families that could not be trusted; where loved ones cause harm or disappear; where no one can be relied upon and where emotional and physical violence was commonplace, the 'anti-group' prevailed, and the group was unable to progress from disparaging and denigrating itself.

Despite this, the group was able to meet for a final session, and consequently the neglect and abandonment of the women's early years was not explicitly enacted. The session took place as planned, perhaps demonstrating to the women, and to myself, that a 'good ending' can itself be seen as a significant achievement. The importance of realistic expectations, and the recognition that small accomplishments have meaning, should not be underestimated in exacting circumstances where, as Nicolas Sarra concedes, 'Sometimes it is not possible to think in a group or do anything apart from survive the experience' (1998, p. 81).

MENTALISATION BASED ART THERAPY GROUP

Mentalisation based therapy (MBT) was conceived by Antony Bateman and Peter Fonagy (2006) specifically to work with individuals with a diagnosis of borderline personality disorder (BPD). Personality disorder as a mental health concept remains contentious, but is endemic in the female prison estate, with in excess of 60% of women meeting the criteria for diagnosis (NOMS, 2015). This in itself is symbolic of the condemnatory and hostile medical hypotheses women assume (Eastwood, 2012), increasingly evident as BPD comes to be seen, more compassionately, as complex post-traumatic stress disorder. MBT has become a popular treatment model within the NHS, perhaps in part because it is a medium-term, manualised therapy and initial training can be completed in just a few days, and also because in a climate that prioritises evidence-based practice, MBT has been researched quantitatively through a number of random controlled trials (Bateman and Fonagy, 2009).

In this milieu of 'evidence-based' treatments and collaborative practice, I felt under pressure from the organisation to offer a group in partnership with the prison drug strategy service. I was informed by the healthcare manager that this should attend to the needs of women with a 'dual diagnosis'; the co-occurrence for an individual of a substance use disorder and a psychiatric disorder. Inevitably, this included many women with traits or a diagnosis of BPD. Thus, I developed the Mentalisation Based Art Therapy (MBAT) group as a structured, integrated, evidence-based and cohesive ten-week programme, which could be easily understood and evaluated for consideration by commissioners. This was a more psycho-social way of working than the earlier groups, which I have previously detailed, practically and theoretically, in the context of modified forensic therapy (Collier and Gee, 2015). From a personal perspective, however, by agreeing to create and facilitate a 'manualised' group, I imagined I was surrendering my agency to the management, and becoming more institutionalised and controlled myself; another parallel process alongside the women, whereby I felt I was made to relinquish my own preferences and follow 'orders'. Understanding my countertransference more deeply, I might also recognise that the group I wanted to facilitate – the long-term, psychoanalytically informed art psychotherapy group described earlier – had already proven to be exhausting for me, and difficult for the women to use; whilst the MBAT group came to be well regarded by the mental health team. This revealed to me how I might resist what others want, and feel compelled to continue with my own preference, even when it might be difficult or damaging; a demonstration perhaps of my identification with the prisoners and the ubiquity of the repetition compulsion (Freud, 1920). Emotional responses occur however much personal psychotherapy or training we undertake, and, as therapists, we should be aware of how unconscious feelings and actions influence our decision making. Thus, my ambivalence about the MBAT group rested, in part perhaps, on my unconscious compulsion not to take the easy option but to feel that the work must be as challenging for me as for the women in the group, reflecting my own familial dynamics. Conversely, I have wondered retrospectively if MBAT was accepted and referred to by colleagues because it was straightforward to understand, and also had an easily discernible name. Groups of all types seem to be valued more in institutions when they have a memorable or appealing title or acronym, and thrive when there are enough resources to publicise effectively. This can be seen as a clear indicator of commercial strategies at work in healthcare and criminal justice settings, and also illustrative of the wish to disavow work that is difficult to comprehend, as it may remind us of what we do not know, and thus our own vulnerability.

Nevertheless, despite my own resistance, I worked hard to make a containing space. Having struggled to facilitate the earlier groups by myself, I felt supported by working alongside my co-facilitator, a thoughtful and consistent drug strategy manager who took an active interest in the art psychotherapy process. Conducting the group as a couple allowed us to model a 'good enough' relationship; demonstrating together the potential for taking creative risks, offering mutual support, turn taking and negotiation. With two facilitators, a strength of the group became its capacity to hold both positive and negative phenomena while maintaining the boundaries and safety of the prisoners in the space. Nevertheless, an overriding similarity across all the work was the depiction of hostile environments: internal and external; symbolic and concrete; conscious and unconscious. These images often appeared in response to the session themes, which included difference, self, relationships, emotions, environment and safe space. As the women attempted to portray their experiences and expectations, metaphors for their hostile familial and social circumstances starkly emerged.

In one session, where time was given for the women to make an image together of their own choosing, their collaborative work represented what they described as the 'perfect place'. Consciously intended to evoke pleasure, even envy, it revealed on closer inspection an environment inhospitable for human life: exposure to searing sun, no shelter, alcohol but no fresh water or food, no means of egress, and as materialised repeatedly in the art work, no other people – the intergenerational inadequacy of the women's interpersonal relationships conspicuous in their absence. During the group discussion, the three women who had worked on the image together were astonished to see the danger and deprivation they had confused with paradise. This observation allowed them to reflect on the way they romanticised their chaotic lifestyles and idealised their neglectful, violent relationships so as to survive the abuse and adversity. It initiated a conversation between them about the reality of the hardships they faced, and the importance of recognising that change was needed.

Artworks where other human figures did emerge would often epitomise the kind of punitive authority the women were all too familiar with, depicting a world of two halves: the vibrant milieu of privilege, power and influence securely on top; the muted experience of deprivation, humiliation and poverty supplicant below; the woman's thoughts and words, illustrated as speech bubbles, emptily wafting, unheard, out of the frame (Figure 8.1).

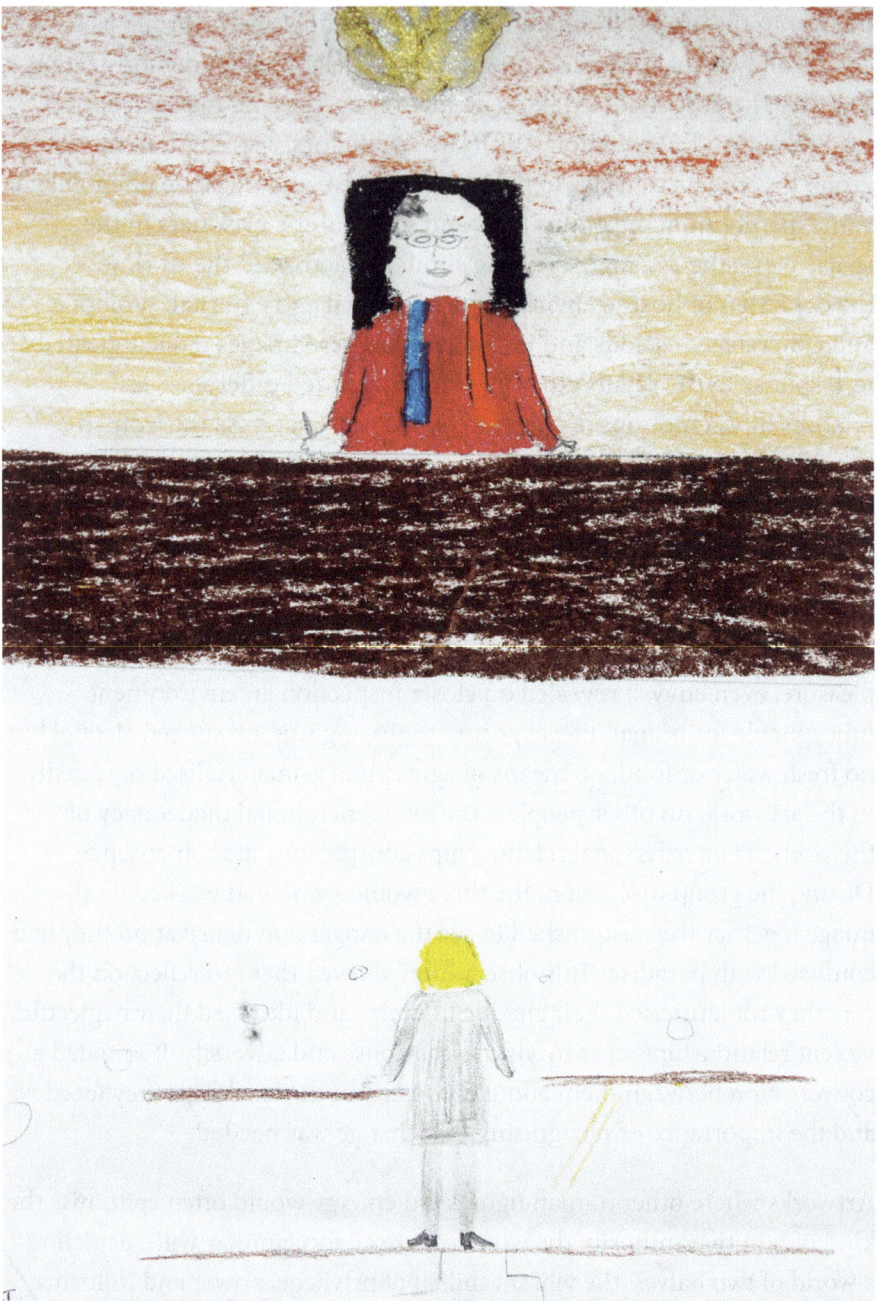

Figure 8.1 *'A world of two halves'. Artwork made by a group member.*

In the imagery, the consequence of such futile interpersonal encounters determined a monochromatic reality of grief, loss and isolation, simultaneously brutal and barren and illustrating the dichotomy of impenetrability and containment provided by the prison walls. The woman who made this drawing (Figure 8.2) reflected that while she had sketched herself, head in hands, with a fragile pencil line, she had represented the cell bars using a permanent marker; stronger and more durable than her. This simple image prompted discussion in the group about emotional defences, the internal prisons we make for ourselves, how powerful they are, and how concrete they may become when left unacknowledged.

Despite my ambivalence about facilitating such directive sessions, the MBAT group seemed to offer the women a glimpse into their inner lives, and perhaps the opportunity to understand their experiences and the origins of their anguish. The tangible framework of the structured sessions seemed to contain some of the anxiety around tolerating uncertainty; the aims and expectations were clear and realistic; and the women were able to focus on their own and others' emotional responses to the imagery.

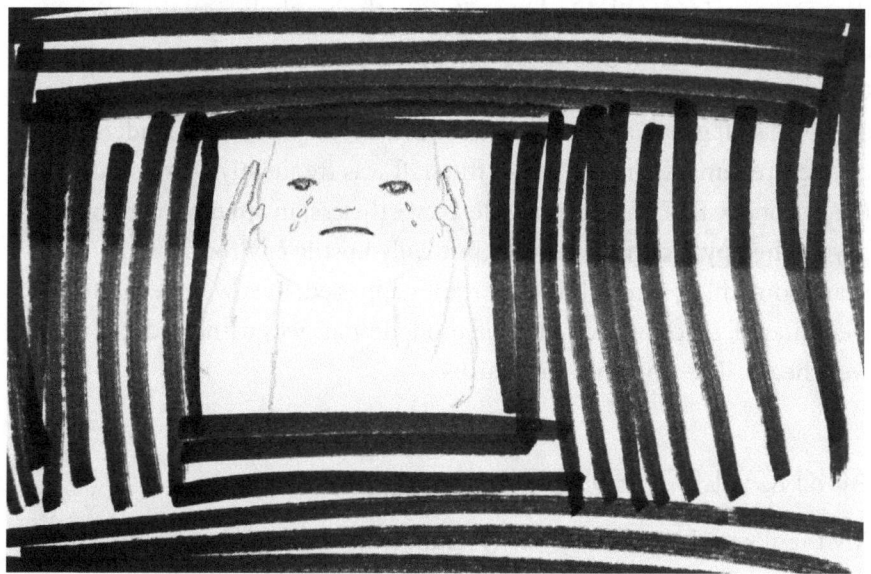

Figure 8.2 'Prison Cell'. Artwork made by a group member.

CONCLUSION

It was perhaps inevitable that having found a way of working that seemed both meaningful and manageable, the possibility of further group provision in the prison was terminated. This was a consequence of the government closing the institution; a cynical and disingenuous act of prison 'reform' that impacted the welfare of the women and their families for the benefit of ill-considered and hostile politics (Stewart and Collier, 2019). While the MBAT group succeeded in giving the women a safe space and a voice – 'That room was my safety net', declared one prisoner – this chapter has not attempted to portray art psychotherapy groups in a female prison as a panacea for extricating 'hope' or 'recovery' from women whose lives are characterised by deprivation, poverty, prejudice and trauma. Rather, it offers a realistic conclusion that effective group psychotherapy is exceptionally difficult to conduct with marginalised people whose impoverished internal world is mirrored in the environments around them. While analytically informed psychodynamic groups can succeed in prison, there must be an institutional investment in this treatment as a shared task between the prison regime of physical security and the psychological therapies objective of prioritising emotional security. Prisons based on Therapeutic Community principles may support a strong enough investment between a diverse staff group and prisoners to sustain the work. In an underfunded city centre remand prison, where the staff was frequently as traumatised as the prisoners, this was not possible. Nevertheless, in attempting to offer art psychotherapy groups in this exceptionally hostile environment, over the years, something simple but important happened: lives were seen; stories were shared; emotions were understood; despair was witnessed and women were heard. The women were heard.

ACKNOWLEDGEMENTS

My thanks to the women at HMP Holloway who had the courage to attend the art psychotherapy groups described in this chapter and to the individuals who consented to their images being shared.

REFERENCES

Bateman, A.W. and Fonagy, P. (2006). Mechanism of change in mentalization based treatment of borderline personality disorder. *Journal of Clinical Psychology*, 62(4), pp. 411–430.

Bateman, A.W. and Fonagy, P. (2009). Randomized controlled trial of outpatient mentalization-based treatment versus structured clinical management for borderline personality disorder. *American Journal of Psychiatry*, 166(12), pp. 1355–1364.

Blake, W. (1794). 'Infant Sorrow'. In: Songs of Innocence and of Experience in *The Portable Blake*, 1974 ed., New York: The Viking Press. First published 1946.

Carlen, P. (2012). Women's imprisonment: An introduction to the Bangkok Rules. *Observatorio del Sistema Penal y los Derechos Humanos*, Universidad de Barcelona, 3, pp. 148–157.

Collier, J. (2015). 3 Man Unlock: Out of sight out of mind. Art Psychotherapy with a woman with severe personality disorder in prison. *Psychoanalytic Psychotherapy*, 29(3), pp. 243–261.

Collier, J. (2019a). Trauma, Art and the 'Borderspace': Working with Unconscious Re-Enactments. In: Stewart, P. and Collier, J. (eds), *The End of the Sentence: The Future of Psychotherapy with Female Offenders*. 1st ed., London: Routledge, pp. 164–182.

Collier, J. (2019b). Cover Stories: Art Psychotherapy with Mothers in Prison Who Have Killed or Harmed Their Children. In: Foster, A. (ed.), *Mothers Accused and Abused: Breaking Cycles of Neglect*. 1st ed., London: Routledge, pp. 96–111.

Collier, J. and Gee, J. (2015). Modifying Therapies: Female Offenders with Personality Disorders. In: Jones, P. (ed.), *Interventions in Criminal Justice: A Handbook for Counsellors and Therapists Working in the Criminal Justice System Volume 2*. 1st ed., Brighton: Pavilion, pp. 75–93.

Cox, J. and Sacks-Jones, K. (2017). 'Double disadvantage: The experiences of Black, Asian and Minority Ethnic women in the criminal justice system'. Agenda Alliance for women and girls at risk. Available at: https://weareagenda.org/wp-content/uploads/2017/03/Double-disadvantage-FINAL.pdf [Accessed 27 January 2021].

Crenshaw, K. (1989). Demarginalizing the intersection of race and sex: A Black feminist critique of antidiscrimination doctrine, feminist theory and antiracist politics. *University of Chicago Legal Forum*, (1), pp. 8. Available at: http://chicagounbound.uchicago.edu/uclf/vol1989/iss1/8 [Accessed 27 January 2021].

Crenshaw, K. (2013). From private violence to mass incarceration: Thinking intersectionally about women, race and social control. *Journal of Scholarly Perspectives*, 9(0), pp. 23–37.

Eastwood, C. (2012). Art therapy with women with borderline personality disorder: A feminist perspective. *International Journal of Art Therapy*, 17(3), pp. 98–114.

Fine, C. (2018). *Testosterone Rex: Unmaking the Myths of Our Gendered Minds*. London: Icon Books.

Foucault, M. (1979). *Discipline and Punish: The Birth of Prison*. 1st ed., Middlesex, England: Penguin Books.

Foulkes, S.H. (1948). *Introduction to Group-Analytic Psychotherapy*. London: Heinemann. Reprinted London: Karnac, 1983.

Freud, S. (1920). *Beyond the Pleasure Principle*. Standard edition. Volume 18. London: Hogarth, pp. 7–65.

Klein, M. (1946). Notes on Some Schizoid Mechanisms. In: *Envy and Gratitude and Other Works 1946–1963*. London: Hogarth Press and the Institute of Psycho-Analysis (published 1975).

Macintyre, D. (2011). 'Major on crime: "Condemn more, understand less"'. *The Independent*, 22 October [online]. Available at: https://www.independent.co.uk/news/major-on-crime-condemn-more-understand-less-1474470.html [Accessed 27 January 2021].

Maynard, K. (2018). To be Black. To be a Woman. Can dramatherapy help Black women to discover their true self despite racial and gender oppression? *Dramatherapy*, 39(1), pp. 31–48.

Medlicott, D. (2007). Women in Prison. In: Jewkes, Y. (ed.), *Handbook on Prisons*. Devon: Willan Publishing, pp. 245–267.

Nitsun, M. (1991). The anti-group: Destructive forces in the group and their therapeutic potential. *Group Analysis*, 24, pp. 7–20

NOMS; National Offender Management Services (2015). *Working with Personality Disorders: A Practitioners Guide*. Available at: https://www.england.nhs.uk/commissioning/wp-content/uploads/sites/12/2015/10/work-offndrs-persnlty-disorder-oct15.pdf [Accessed 27 January 2021].

Prison Reform Trust (2018). 'Nineteen in 20 children forced to leave home when mum goes to jail' [online]. Available at: http://www.prisonreformtrust.org.uk/PressPolicy/News/vw/1/ItemID/545 [Accessed 27 January 2021].

Ruszczynski, S. (2012). What Makes a Setting Secure? In: Adlam, J., Aiyegbusi, A., Kleinot, P., Motz, A. and Scanlon, C. (eds), *The Therapeutic Milieu under Fire: Security and Insecurity in Forensic Mental Health*. 1st ed., London and Philadelphia: Jessica Kingsley Publishers, pp. 200–211.

Sarra, N. (1998). Connection and Disconnection in the Art Therapy Group: Working with Forensic Patients in Acute States on a Locked Ward. In: Skaife, S. and Huet, V. (eds), *Art Psychotherapy Groups: Between Pictures and Words*. 1st ed., London: Routledge, pp. 69–87.

Scanlon, C. (2012). The Traumatised-Organisation-in-the-Mind: Opening up Space for Difficult Conversations in Difficult Places. In: Adlam, J., Aiyegbusi, A., Kleinot, P., Motz, A. and Scanlon, C. (eds), *The Therapeutic Milieu under Fire: Security and Insecurity in Forensic Mental Health*. 1st ed., London and Philadelphia: Jessica Kingsley Publishers, pp. 212–228.

Scott, D. (2007). The Changing Face of the English Prison: A Critical Review of the Aims of Imprisonment. In: Jewkes, Y. (ed.), *Handbook on Prisons*. Devon: Willan Publishing, pp. 49–72.

Smart, C. (1976). *Women, Crime and Criminology: A Feminist Critique*. London: Routledge and Kegan Paul.

Soothill, K. (2007). Prison Histories and Competing Audiences, 1776–1966. In: Jewkes, Y. (ed.), *Handbook on Prisons*. Devon: Willan Publishing, pp. 27–48.

Stewart, P. and Collier, J. (eds) (2019). *The End of the Sentence: The Future of Psychotherapy with Female Offenders*. Abingdon and New York: Routledge.

Williams, K., Papadopoulou, V. and Booth, N. (2012). Results from the Surveying Prisoner Crime Reduction (SPCR) longitudinal cohort study of prisoners. *Ministry of Justice Analytical Services Ministry of Justice Research Series 4/12*.

Women in Prison (n.d.) Available at: https://www.womeninprison.org.uk/about/key-facts

Woolf, H. (1991). *Prison Disturbances April 1990: Report of an Inquiry*. London: HMSO.

Yalom, I.D. (1975). *The Theory and Practice of Group Psychotherapy*. 1st ed., New York: Basic Books.

CHAPTER NINE

Protested space
Artworks made in a therapeutic art studio under threat from cuts

Helen Omand

DOI: 10.4324/9781003107408-12

Art has a rich history as an agent of protest. This chapter will consider how artworks, made in a therapeutic art studio, were radical acts of protest for the group. These artworks were made in response to the partial closure of the service due to austerity-driven funding cuts and a sense of wider political and social injustice. In the chapter I examine the tension I felt as an art therapist between an initial wish to protect and shield the group from knowing the truth about the financial pressures (the studio as a 'protected space') and a desire to go with the potential for empowerment that knowing the worst, and becoming part of a joined-up community response to the closures, might provide. The studio became a 'protested space' in which art was an active agent. Viewed like this the art illuminates the hierarchical tensions within the therapy space during this time of crisis, where the more radical community-based ethos of the studio seemed under threat of erosion by powerful social, economic and political forces, and felt difficult to maintain. The art can be seen as giving form to this ethos.

Some of the artworks discussed here were put up on the studio wall by members during this time as a deliberate protest against the closures. Others were left out on easels or shelves from week to week, or shared and hidden away, or even exhibited in public. From my discussions with the artists, I started to consider that these artworks, with their often-overt political subject matter, had agency as a voice of dissent. It seemed to me that the images had a life in the studio space and contributed to the experience of this particular period, when the impact of social, political and economic forces threatened the studio's survival.

Seven images from studio artists are presented here alongside their words about their images. This chapter seeks to think about the role these images may have had for the wider studio group at this time, particularly as acts of protest. I refer in this chapter to the 'community' of the whole organisation, but of course there are many differences, intersections of identities and power relationships within this. I am conscious of not being able to speak for the whole therapy team, or an imagined homogenous community, a 'we'. Instead this chapter is a personal and subjective attempt to make meaning from images, words and memories of this particular time in the studio's history.

ORGANISATIONAL CONTEXT

The Human Arts Studio[1] is for adults experiencing a range of enduring mental health difficulties, for example psychosis of one kind or another, or profound struggles with relationships. Most people have been in the mental health system for some time. The studio was founded on the radical principles of therapeutic communities, the anti-psychiatry movement, R.D. Laing and the Philadelphia Association. Service users are called 'members' to reflect this ethos. Certain principles remain decades on: the community forum, where all have a say in the running of the studio; the involvement of studio members in decision making; the emphasis on people rather than diagnoses that may pathologise; and the attempt to lessen the hierarchy of therapist/client. Therapists make art and exhibit work alongside members in regular exhibitions. The shared struggle with creative processes may contribute to a flattening of the hierarchy, with therapists on more equal ground with members. For example, some members may be more accomplished artists in particular mediums, and there is much sharing of knowledge in the group. I have attended workshops that members have given for the studio community. Additionally, with making art and with having long contact hours, more aspects of the therapist as a complex individual are seen.

The equality of 'we are all artists together' exists on some levels, yet at the same time can be somewhat idealised, as, of course, there are all sorts of hierarchies and differences in the group. The current organisational structure is hierarchical: a management level and their administrative team; the art therapists, students and volunteers; and members. Monthly team meetings include all levels of the organisation, including member representatives. To avoid confusion for the purposes of this chapter, I will call the art therapists 'therapists', the management and administration 'management' and the wider membership 'members', or in the context of their artwork, 'artists'.

The studio opened most days of the week 10am–5pm, the space overseen by two co-therapists on each day. Each day hosts a consistent group

---

1 The organisation has been anonymised.

of members who come and go as they wish during the day. Some stay a whole day, others manage less. The space is a working art studio, crowded, rich and stimulating, crammed with easels, ceramics equipment, folders, piles of canvases and work left drying. There is a kitchen and CD player. In my experience, long-term members care deeply about this environment and contribute to it, bringing in shared food, art donations or music to play.

EVENTS LEADING UP TO THE CLOSURES

The studio is unusual in offering long-term support and community to its members in a climate in which cheaper, short-term therapy, CBT, and tick box recovery plans are dominant. As government mental health funding reduced year on year, local authority payments that had historically funded individual members to attend the studio increasingly dried up, despite willingness of mental health teams on the ground to refer. This affected the studio's income and threatened the sustainability of surviving on local authority payments. Meanwhile, punitive government disability benefit reassessment schemes increased member anxiety. The impact of austerity policies was felt in ever-increasing cuts. Studio management regularly mooted closing days, which would result in established groups shutting and jobs being lost. There were splits over the differing priorities of management and therapists as to whether closures were needed. Management, pragmatically, wanted to diversify our approach to increase economic sustainability, whereas therapists focused on the detrimental effects of the reduction in the service.

Around this time, management and therapists held several team meetings without member representatives; we discussed studio finances and the real threat of day closures, and I remember worrying, like others, that these discussions might be overwhelming for members. With hindsight, the exclusion of members from these meetings seemed to reassert hierarchy. I felt caught up in the dilemma of how far we should share financial problems with members, and how far we should contain the anxiety amongst staff until we were more certain about the outcome. However, we did not want to patronise members and there was the possibility that some would want to voice opposition and take action. Therapists tried to hold the uncertainty at this time. In a strange parallel, during this period the physical environment also started to be gradually eroded; the building that housed the studio was emptied for renovation by developers. We remained clinging on like a last bastion as facilities and lifts were stripped out. There was a feeling of huddling against the storm.

The following monthly meeting was attended by member representatives and staff. Management announced its decision to members and therapists at the same time to cut the service by over a third, and in a matter of weeks. The impact was palpable, leaving us momentarily lost for words. A community that had weathered the storms of decades went into a sort of shock. Long established day groups were to be closed, losing several therapist positions.

Emergency meetings were held by members and therapists to ascertain possible action plans. Disbelief was followed by anger and a call to action from members. This was a period of upset and distress, but also, I felt, one of solidarity between members and therapists. Members got together to campaign and write letters, and therapists formed proposals for alternative financial options. The endless meetings and negotiation of co-operative working took its toll on all, as did the split between management and the therapists and members.

Our collective efforts were in vain and reality hit – we had not stopped the closures. Therapists faced the prospect of ending their groups and, if they wanted to stay on in the organisation, being re-interviewed for the remaining jobs. Some members found it too painful to come in at all and detached from the studio. Members who chose to stay were amalgamated into existing groups. As a community we started the uncomfortable process of moving forward.

ARTIST IMAGES AND TEXT

The following images were chosen after discussion with each member. The accompanying words are extracts from recorded conversations which I co-edited with each member. Members chose to use their real names to credit authorship of both artwork and words, which is in the studio's ethos of promoting the development of artistic identity. Artwork is regularly exhibited under people's names. Each artist therefore had to feel sure that they were happy for their work and statement to be in the public domain. The artworks are presented here in chronological order of their making.

'SGT MAYBOT'S LONELY HEARTS CLUBBED BANNED' BY JAKE SUMMER (FIGURE 9.1)

The large canvas painting of Trump and May had an ongoing presence in the studio in the year prior to the cuts. Summer says:

> It reflects that period when Theresa May was Prime Minister, after Donald Trump was declared President. It was inspired by May 'holding hands' with Trump. There is the sense of a couple presiding over a scene of desolation. There is an absence of love and happiness. A group of far-right figures, emulating a zombie takeover, are surrounding a girl in a burka, like bloodhounds. The husk-like structure gives a sense of something arising from the ashes, from all this apocalypse. I think the terrible image of Grenfell tower was somewhere in there as an influence.
>
> There is a characterisation of a harsh uncaring couple – certainly Trump makes no indication that he actually cares for the world. He denies all very real problems like climate change. May was very willing to side with Trump, little good that it did her. It was a very tragic relationship, which is reflected in the painting, but let's not waste our tears on the architect of the 'hostile environment' and someone who was all too complicit in brutal austerity.

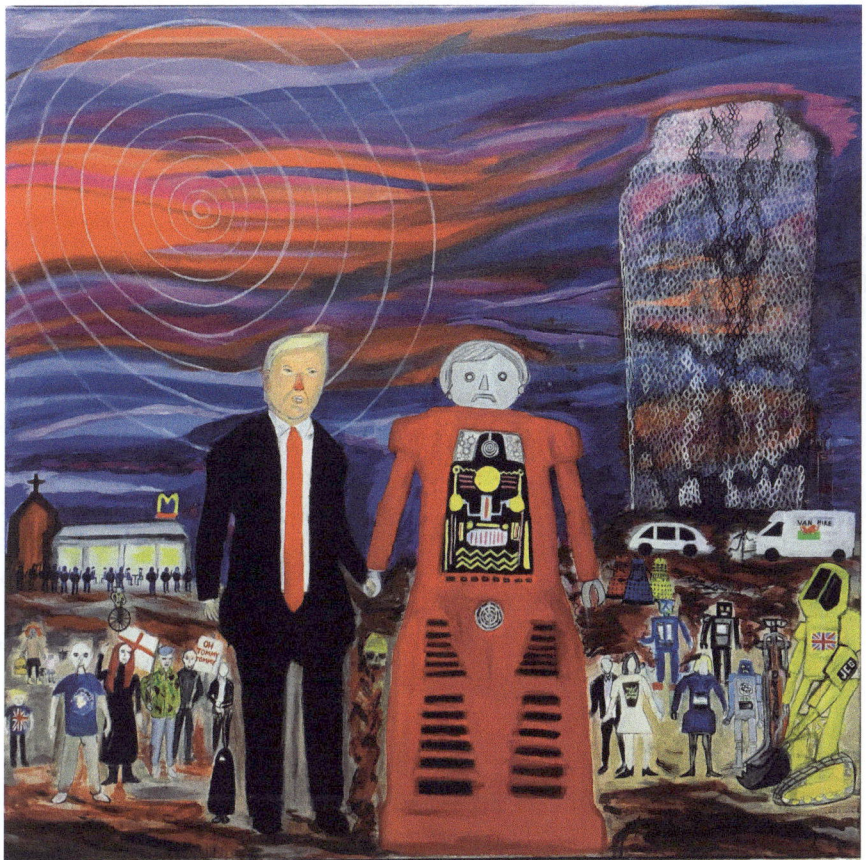

Figure 9.1 *'Sgt Maybot's lonely hearts clubbed banned' by Jake Summer. Oil on canvas.*

There's billions of pounds spent on nuclear weapons, while getting access to NHS mental health support is nearly impossible. Punitive welfare reforms have left people actually dying from hunger. The poor are dying under the Tory government. Warnings are given; if you cut this far, it will kill people. But who cares when you're poor? I live in a constant state of anxiety, magnified by the rhetoric of austerity. Art can be a form of protest because we are often disempowered: art is a means of reflecting our disenfranchisement. Sometimes when you see an artwork or you hear a good song – it doesn't have to be something political necessarily – but speaking about what's upsetting you in the world, it means a lot that somebody did that. On Donald Trump's official visit last year his helicopter flight route happened to be right over the studio. I brought my painting out onto the top balcony with a sign I made saying 'No, Donald, no'.

'AUSTERI-TEA' BY RACHEL ROWAN OLIVE (FIGURE 9.2)

Rowan Olive says:

It's about the pattern of what's happened since my breakdown, all the way through my time in the system, over and over again. I was at a day hospital when they had just lost their funding and were changing their model because of that – making everything really short and time-limited and pushing people out as quickly as possible. Crisis house stays are really short-term and I was being told to ask for help, but then there just wasn't anything there. It was a painful, damaging process.

The way that you're constantly told this is not really what's happening, goes back to the idea of being given piss and being told it's tea – you're told so much of the time that your perceptions are wrong. It gets pushed back onto you. 'If we can't meet your needs, it's because your needs are wrong.' It creates so many probably abusive dynamics that … that's what drives people mad. When all the stuff happened with the threat of studio days closing, it was like, okay, here we fucking go again.

'BREXIT POSTER' BY JAKE SUMMER. INK ON PAPER (FIGURE 9.3)

The 'Brexit poster' is inspired by the cold war era government information programme, Protect and Survive, about nuclear attack. It shows what could potentially happen in the worst-case scenario of a no-deal Brexit.

Underneath the house there's a bunker in which the perfect stiff-upper-lip family – loyalist, rule Britannia, never question the government, Brexit all the way – they're ready … well, they think they're ready, in their bunker. They've stockpiled water, food, medicine, toiletries, and all the essential items that one would need to see through

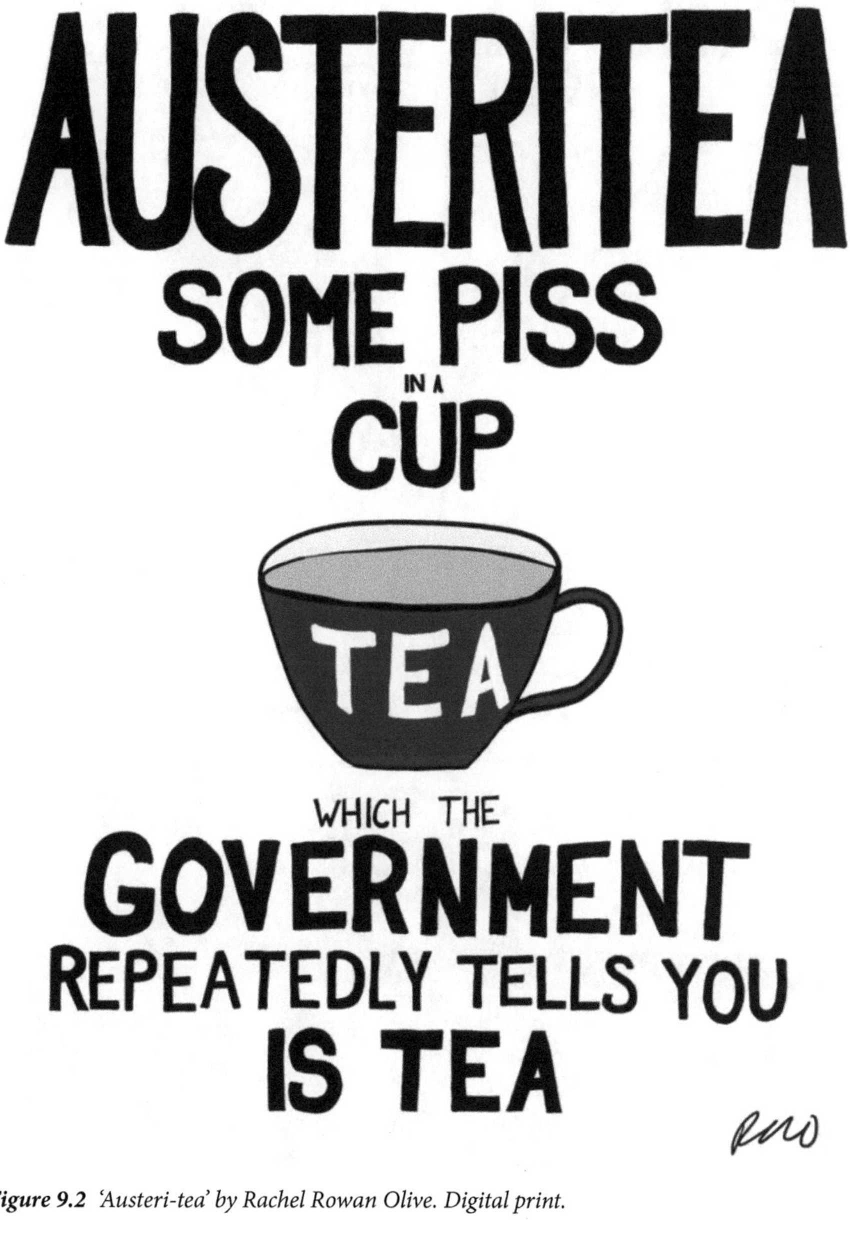

Figure 9.2 *'Austeri-tea' by Rachel Rowan Olive. Digital print.*

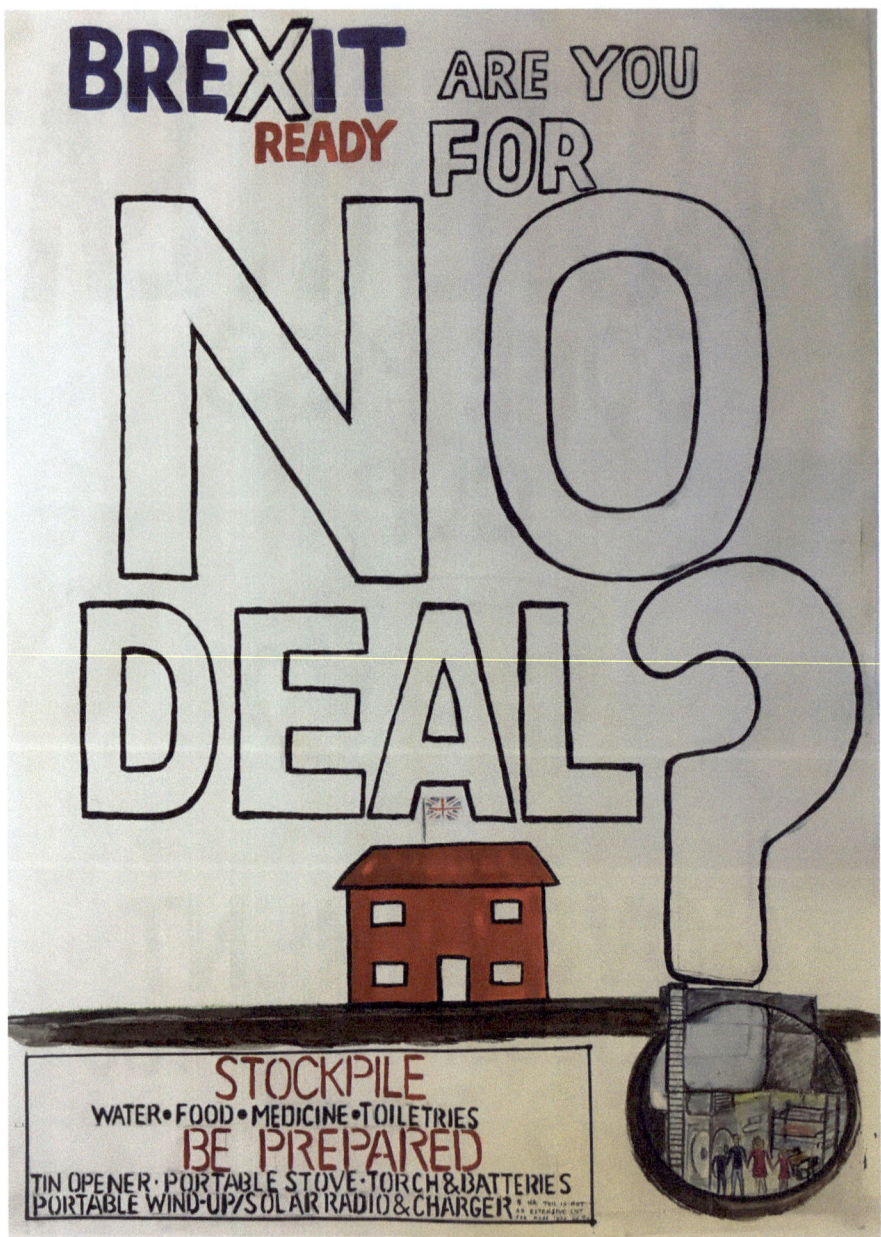

Figure 9.3 *'Brexit poster' by Jake Summer. Ink on paper.*

the disaster. The image is really informed by ... kind of an impending sense of doom, Armageddon, that the Brexit no-deal scenario poses.

'GRAYSON PERRY' BY TORIA LAMB (FIGURE 9.4)

Artist Toria Lamb made this work as the closures were announced.

It was a lot of fear. Everybody was frightened that they might lose this space altogether – that the studio might close. The fear is that you might lose the service that you really need. I feel secure here. It's a place where the vulnerable come when their, you know, their life is falling apart and they're trying to put it back together. So, I did a picture of Grayson Perry – I just felt that somebody needed to be sticking up for us.

I asked, why Grayson Perry?

I just really like Grayson Perry. He does a lot of stuff, art stuff. He looks at society and he seems to take a sort of ... a look, and he seems to

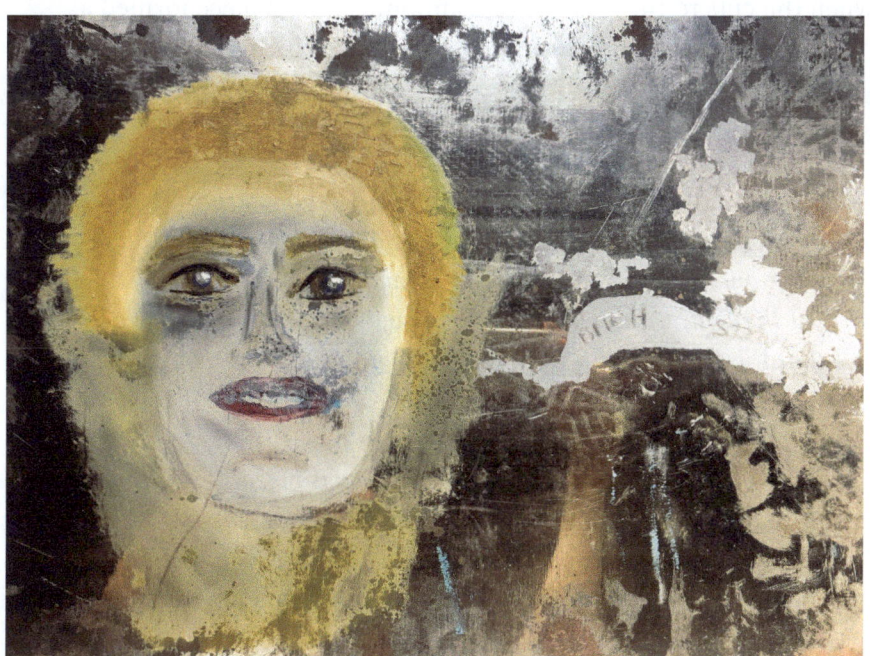

Figure 9.4 *'Grayson Perry' by Toria Lamb. Paint on mirror.*

care about political things and care about people. I don't know whether
he does or not, but he seems to. I thought he'd be a good role model.
A floating head. He's saying some horrible words directed towards
management – I was frightened to say them myself. They're cutting
words and I carved them in. It's faint, I suppose because anger is
frightening to me.

Maybe my anger was misdirected. You don't know who's responsible.
Maybe it's wider political, you know, austerity. The words could
go anywhere … to anybody in a position of power, who are taking
advantage. It was a really difficult time. The inequality goes against the
community spirit of the studio. I wanted someone like Grayson Perry to
step in.

'WOUNDED BEAR' BY ANDREW MEAD (FIGURE 9.5)

Figure 9.5, 'Wounded Bear' by Andrew Mead, began a series of work
that was posted up on the walls of the main studio space as protest
when the cuts to the service were announced. The piece formed a
backdrop to studio life during these months, which included whole
group forums, team meetings and supervisions all happening in the
space. Mead says:

It was using the walls to exhibit our work – but angry work related to
the closures. There was a political element to it, a protest. And it kind of
grew, once I'd put the Wounded bear up.

I thought 'wounded bear' was a good phrase. It occurred to me
that the studio was a wounded bear and that we're not going to give
in lightly. If you back a wounded bear into a corner, it comes out
fighting. It goes vicious. The idea of wounds, cuts, is of something
that has been, damaged I guess. The bear is bleeding. Perhaps
from his mouth, or maybe he's spitting blood or spitting nails. He's
probably bleeding internally as well. I think I saw myself as part of
the studio and therefore part of the image of the wounded bear. It
all mashed into one. I felt we were so messed with that we wanted to
fight.

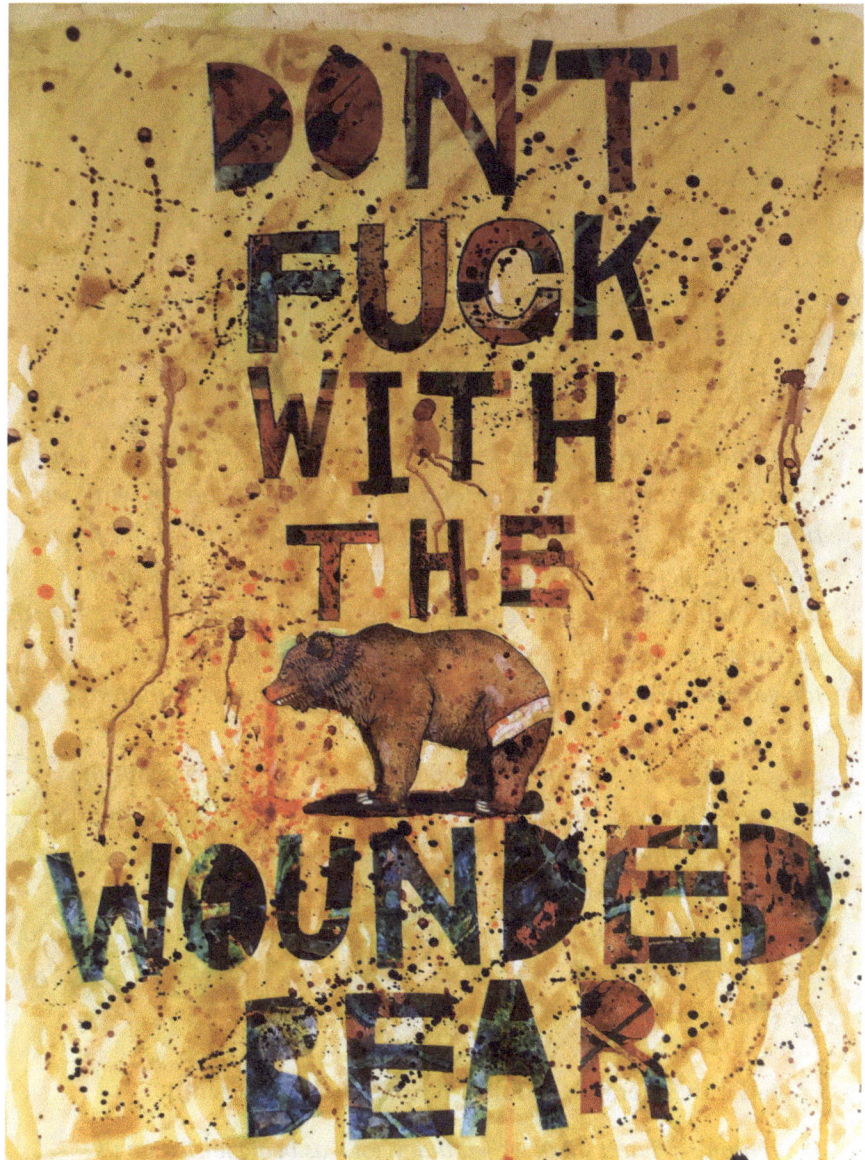

Figure 9.5 *'Wounded Bear' by Andrew Mead. Collage on paper.*

The response from other members was surprisingly positive, the work seemed to channel other people's anger and distress. I was quite nervous about putting it up. I was aware that when we had meetings the Wounded Bear would be behind where the management sat and could be seen by us but not them. I felt it empowered the group and was, sort of, sticking two fingers out behind or something. Solidarity – like looking to a masthead.

Alongside Mead's work, an anonymous contributor had pinned up another sheet of paper with more expletives scrawled on it. Mead also posted up enlarged photocopies of work from his sketchbook. The pieces were based around text, a series of slogans or communications. One of these read 'TOTAL CONTEMPT FOR VULNERABLE LIVES', on collaged paper. Mead says:

It felt quite empowering that I'd done something private that I could expose to the world. I wasn't holding back, various bits of work were tumbling out. And I wasn't showing that it was okay. I think they were quite personal. I mean my emotional background is about being bullied. When you're bullied, there's no communication. If you accede to the bully then you're not answering back or standing up for yourself or something, so maybe that was triggered, that kind of feeling.

'Showing contempt for vulnerable lives' was definitely about the members. The way the cuts were announced didn't acknowledge the impact it might have on individuals. There was a lot of anger targeted towards the management after this, rightly or wrongly, possibly scapegoating. But there were perhaps ways it could have been handled differently. The communication was poor. It felt brutal – 'We're cutting the studio. Thank you for coming. Goodbye'.

I ask Mead if the therapists could have handled it differently.

I'm reminded that, I think we felt that a lot was being foisted on us members to deal with it as opposed to staff taking responsibility of standing up to management decisions. As though members were in the best position to object, like we had more power. Because you (the therapists) were all fairly vulnerable because of the nature of your employment contracts there was the feeling that we were being expected to do more than reasonable because we're the clients. I think it was hard. There was that feeling of not being protected. Maybe it was good that we had to write letters and take it on. Maybe that was empowering. But exposing. Less comfortable.

'REUSABLE PROTEST PLACARD' BY RACHEL ROWAN OLIVE (FIGURE 9.6)

There's so much to protest, just have a reusable one. It just saves time these days. I made postcards of this image, and I feel tempted to just keep one in my bag at all times to bring out if someone pisses me off (laughs). Usually the people who find my art funniest are people who've been in similar situations. People in most of the spaces that I am in are subject to multiple marginalisation and oppressions, and so they get the humour. It's a nice side effect if it challenges the way clinicians and professionals see you, but that's not really what it's for, it's for me and my friends.

'MYSTIC MENEN, THE EMPRESS OF ETHIOPIA, HER IMPERIAL MAJESTY' BY RSJ (FIGURE 9.7)

The final image is by artist RSJ and was made some months later in the aftermath of the changes. It stuck in my mind particularly as RSJ had been completely absent from the studio since the closures. He arrived back unexpectedly and met, for the first time, the newly amalgamated group he had been allocated to. He immediately painted an image, 'Mystic Menen, the Empress of Ethiopia, Her Imperial Majesty'. RSJ says about his image:

That was the first piece of the year, and it was delayed because of my absence from the studio. It's from a photograph where I thought she looked very mystical, she had a power. It gives her a spiritual feeling like she is being lifted up … an honourable woman. That circle looks like some kind of platform almost, like a mystical platform. She's floating. And then, it also looks like the sun in another way. So, hope for brightness, protection.

The studio causes you to look within yourself for the answers to whatever you're going through. Because I made it on my first day back, this piece is like it was from two different worlds. Actually – when you

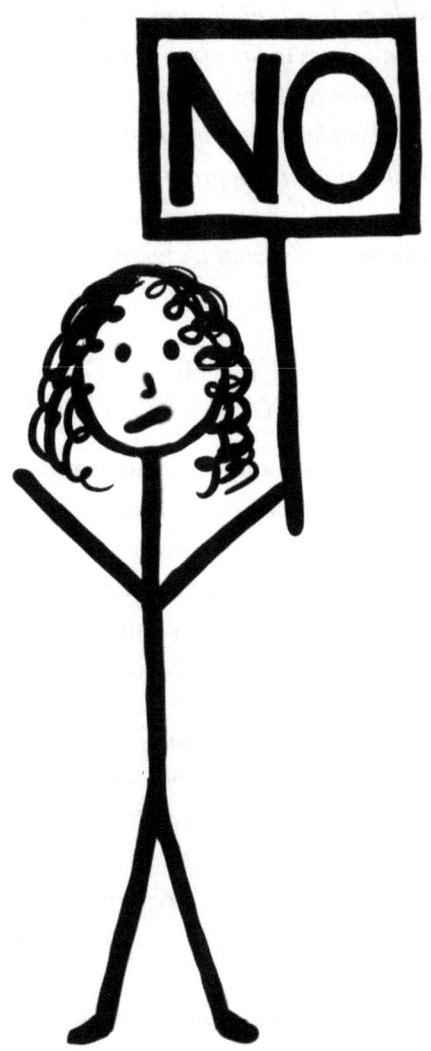

Figure 9.6 *'Reusable protest placard' by Rachel Rowan Olive. Digital print.*

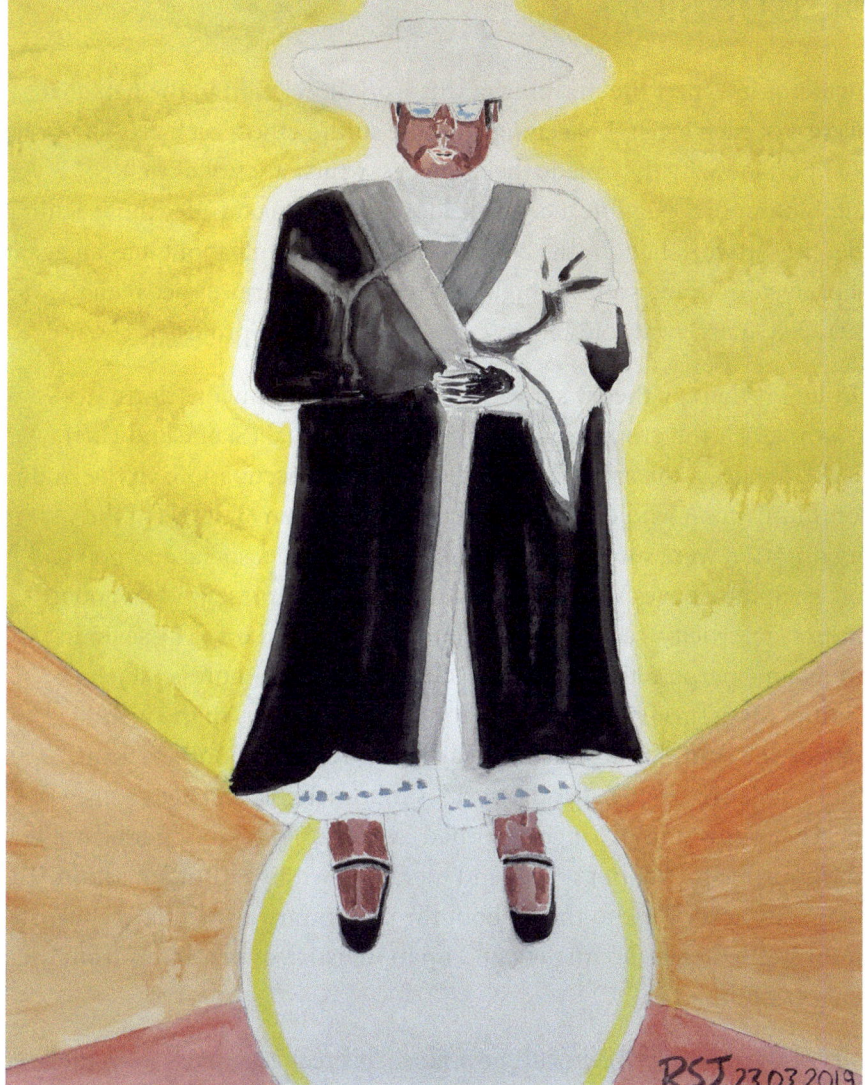

Figure 9.7 *'Mystic Menen, the Empress of Ethiopia, Her Imperial Majesty' by RSJ. Acrylic on canvas.*

look at it, you don't see the war I had been going through. Simplistic –
there's a simplicity about it; the hopeful protective elements rather
than the complicated, destructive elements. It's important to do art
that reflects humanity, especially in inhumane times, so people can
remember what humanity is.

DISCUSSION

I will not interpret the meaning of this work in relation to the personal history of each artist. In keeping with the studio ethos, each artist is 'expert' on why they made these images, which are full of rich autobiographical significance. Instead, I'm going to consider the meaning that this artwork had for the community, and to think about it as an agent of protest. In doing so I will highlight the tension it raises between the therapist's perceived role as 'protector' and as fellow 'protester'.

Group art therapy theory shows artworks will have unconscious meanings for the group as well as for the individual (Skaife and Huet, 1998). I suggest the artworks here reflect the preoccupations of the studio community as a whole at this particular time, when all levels of the organisation were subject to destabilising economic, social and political forces. Some images show powerful figures who represent ideas about fairness or cruelty, care or neglect, and who are held up to be saviours, protectors, perpetrators or villains; Grayson Perry, Empress Menen, Trump, May. The art seems to mirror the split feelings in the world outside the studio, where divisions between rich and poor feel acute, individuals are atomised and 'Brexit' is imminent. The images convey themes of power used for good or bad by authority figures, perhaps also reflecting feelings about power and hierarchy within the organisation. The images prompted me to think about the community's wish for scapegoats or for individuals who might stand up to injustice or protect us from the horrors of the world.

Part of the difficulty I felt with how far to 'protect' members from the anxiety of the truth about financial problems may stem from tensions in how therapeutic work in studios has been conceptualised. For example, to what extent are therapists seen as symbolic parental caregivers, and how far is the group, or community, seen as empowering itself? In recent decades studios in inpatient settings have been thought of as holding environments by art therapists, using objects relations theory. The space, which is provided by the therapist, has been regarded as having a maternal holding or containing function (Brown, 2008, Killick,

2000, Deco, 1998). I have previously found this theoretical frame useful, perhaps like other art therapists, in response to the fragmentary feeling of working with psychosis where a concrete, and symbolic, holding space feels so necessary. Within this framework the sudden shutting down of the therapeutic space could be experienced as a catastrophic withdrawal of holding, with the therapist potentially in the role of neglectful or failing caregiver. This emphasises a more dyadic hierarchical relationship than that of a group. There may be a danger here, in the context of a community group, that members could be disempowered by being perceived as the 'vulnerable' ones within this hierarchy. In fact, we are all vulnerable without the support of others in our communities. The wish to hold on to the responsibility for the financial information about the studio may be our defense, as therapists, in the face of unstoppable economic forces and our own distress. Later, when members were protesting about the cuts, artist Andrew Mead observed that the therapy team's lack of contractual rights meant we appeared vulnerable. It may have felt difficult for members to express anger with the therapists who were so obviously affected too, by loss of jobs. There may have been anger at the therapists' lack of agency, which meant that things felt 'foisted' onto members instead, and that ultimately this powerlessness meant therapists had to go along with the cuts to keep their jobs. These feelings and what they represented may not have been explored enough.

Having considered some of the hierarchical tensions that seemed to be present in the artwork for us as a community, I will now suggest a more active role for art as an act of protest. From political posters to acerbic humour and dystopian scenes, the artworks and statements in this chapter are also a critical voice, drawing attention to harsh policies that have cost lives and marginalised sections of society. A body of art therapy literature draws on social critical theory to acknowledge the systemic power injustices that pervade our social systems and impact individuals, and this literature sees art as a force for empowerment (e.g. Huss, 2015, Hogan, 2016, Talwar, 2019). Similarly, the art here is socially engaged and actively political. Jake Summer's images, for example, highlight injustices, and RSJ's image purposefully expresses his views. Artists are subverting, commenting on, giving shape to, and communicating their experiences of the world.

However, the initiatives most often described in that literature (ibid) are usually co-designed with local communities and the art therapist specifically to empower members of their group, and so, by nature, they are directive projects that center around an issue or theme to be explored. Unlike these, the art in this chapter erupted unsolicited in an established, non-directive therapeutic space. Like Toria Lamb's spikey criticism, or Andrew Mead's texts, art here had the subversion of unauthorised, unspoken commentary. The politics of power, hierarchy, inequality and resistance were present, invited or not, in the art. I suggest this is because they were part of the latent ever-present material of the group itself. Here, a non-directive group space enabled this artwork to be brought into being. The display and presence of artworks in the therapeutic space communicated across the weeks and ensured all levels of the organisation would see them.

The work's agency or power can be thought about further. As a communication about the cuts, the wall of slogans in the main space was striking. Positioned by the table used for team meetings, they formed the backdrop to organisational meetings during this period and were impossible for management and therapists to miss. The artwork was a pointed reminder of the departure that we had made from the historic studio ethos of community representation at meetings. 'Total disrespect for vulnerable lives' seems to call into question the values and priorities of studio staff, as accounting and monetisation to keep the service afloat took priority. Certainly, in relation to the art world, there are many examples of work that takes the principles of the artists to those that exclude them, for example, the posters of the Guerilla girls outside gallery entrances voice criticism of suspect practices by the powerful individuals in charge.

Protest art has long been used to create networks of like-minded individuals for the purposes of resistance, and to convey particular causes or messages. In the studio, artworks may also have been a way of bringing studio members together, aligning ideas and forming social consciousness. Rachel Rowan Olive's comic strips do this using subversive shared humour, Andrew Mead's slogans acted as 'a masthead' to rally behind, reminiscent of art made by political activists: murals, pamphlets, posters, interventions and subversions of logos, and signage and zines. Certainly, over this time members initiated a series of meetings from which organised actions emerged in the form of research, letters and petitions against the closures.

Andrew Mead describes how 'the work seemed to channel other people's anger and distress'. Looking at these artworks, the nuclear explosions, expletives and wounded bear bring back for me the raw feelings of the time, a painful and furious outcry. They are also images of violent acts and, of course, protest can be violent. Members and therapists half joked together about a sit in, or refusing to shut. Perhaps there was an idea from members that the therapist's actions did not go far enough, and perhaps we agreed.

Did we the therapists 'fight' for our principles? For example, could we have done more to keep the groups from closing so suddenly? With the precarious positions of the therapists, perhaps members felt it was left to them to protest and be the culture carriers of the radical history of the studio community. The artworks were used in the space in a way that could be seen as giving form to the radical ethos of the studio's founding, an ethos at risk of being eroded by the new paradigm of the marketised health system that brought the funding cuts, and which perpetuates precarious employment.

Brian Haw, an anti-war protester, occupied a tent outside the Houses of Parliament in London for 10 years to bring attention to the UK and US foreign policy in Afghanistan and Iraq. He became synonymous with his violent and hand-painted placards that pointed blame at the government as killers of innocents. These had a visual presence for a decade in parliament square; a constant embodiment of the government's moral duty. He had much public support and, as such, he protested 'for' the wider group. The art here perhaps also communicated something for us therapists, too, that we did not feel able to communicate ourselves.

While writing this I often found it difficult to separate out the therapists' feelings from those of the members; a painful problem embedded in the fact that therapists are both 'with' the members and also, in some ways, partly responsible for the cuts as staff, because at some point we had to go along with them, to accept them and keep our jobs. The dynamics of the power-infused 'therapist/client' dyad, which the original studio ethos had wanted to eradicate, were complex to negotiate in a shared struggle. Equally difficult was to think that the management level of the organisation also felt in an insurmountable position – to keep the studio viable under pressure from changing mental health paradigms and powerful political and economic agendas. Art historian Kester, writing about activist art, concludes that as the concept of community itself is under threat from global capitalism, 'concepts of collective solidarity and community identity have never been more important. It's impossible to underestimate the significance of community as an organizing principle for resistance and political identity ...' (2003, p. 8). I wonder, in these pressing times of cuts and hardship, how there can be more collaborative working in therapeutic spaces. The artwork in this chapter helps generate thoughts about the hierarchical positions we take up in therapeutic spaces in relation to each other. Seen as acts of protest, the art here embodies the struggle of holding on to more egalitarian principles in today's climate.

I would like to thank and acknowledge the members who so generously contributed their images and words to this chapter.

REFERENCES

Brown, C. (2008). Very toxic – Handle with care. Some aspects of the maternal function in art therapy. *International Journal of Art Therapy*, 13(1), pp. 13–24.

Deco, S. (1998). Return to the Open Studio Group: Art Therapy Groups in Acute Psychiatry. In: Skaife, S. and Huet, V. (eds), *Art Psychotherapy Groups: Between Pictures and Words*. 1st ed., London: Routledge, pp. 88–108.

Hogan, S. (2016). *Art Therapy Theories: A Critical Introduction.* 1st ed., Oxen and New York: Routledge.

Huss, E. (2015). *A Theory-Based Approach to Art Therapy.* 1st ed., London and New York: Routledge.

Kester, G. (2003). Beyond the white cube: Activist art and the legacy of the 1960s. Except from Conversation Pieces: Community and Communication in Modern Art. *Public Art Review*, 14(2), pp. 4–11.

Killick, K. (2000). The Art Room as Container in Analytical Art Psychotherapy with Patients in Psychotic States. In: Gilroy, A. and McNeilly G. (eds), *The Changing Shape of Art Therapy*. London and Philadelphia: Jessica Kingsley, pp. 99–114.

Skaife, S. and Huet, V. (1998). Dissonance and Harmony. Theoretical Issues in Art Psychotherapy Groups. In: Skaife, S. and Huet, V. (eds), *Art Psychotherapy Groups: Between Pictures and Words*. 1st ed., East Sussex, USA and Canada: Routledge, pp. 17–45.

Talwar, S. (2018). *Art Therapy for Social Justice: Radical Intersections*. 1st ed., New York and Oxon: Routledge.

CHAPTER TEN

Witnessing the edge
Reflections on co-facilitating a men's art therapy group in a refugee camp in Greece

Emily Hollingsbee and Katie Miller

DOI: 10.4324/9781003107408-13

INTRODUCTION

People seeking asylum can spend years waiting for their application to be processed and a decision to be reached. In some countries refugee camps are set up as temporary living spaces where people remain until they are granted status. During this time they have no legal right to work, cannot travel freely, and have limited access to state services, often relying on support from charities. Claiming asylum leaves people occupying a precarious threshold, and for long periods of time they are neither in nor out of a state. As Daniel Trilling (2018, p. 241) says, 'The definition of "refugee" is political, and its meaning is subject to a constant struggle over who's in and who's out.'

This chapter explores our experiences as two art psychotherapists co-facilitating art therapy groups in a refugee camp in Greece. The work spanned 18 months between 2016 and 2018. The chapter concentrates on the men's art therapy groups, as they were the most attended sessions and became a large focus of the work. We explore our observations, thoughts and feelings about working in this particular environment, and consider our identities as white, British, female art psychotherapists in relation to this work. Through two vignettes we reflect on the systems we were a part of and consider what we witnessed of people living on the edge.

To provide context and ease of reading we will be using the following terms within the chapter: refugee, a person who has been forced to flee their home country due to fear of war and persecution; asylum seeker, a person who has made an application to seek asylum (UNHCR, 2020a); residents, persons living in the refugee camp who may be categorised as either refugee or asylum seeker.

WORKING IN GREECE

Our decision to leave the UK and work in Greece was motivated by both emotional and economic factors that we were experiencing in our country. We had previously worked together as art facilitators with unaccompanied and asylum-seeking young people in the Calais refugee camp known as 'The Jungle' and had a specific interest in working within this area. As we watched the media's often dehumanising portrayal of refugees and asylum seekers, we felt driven to respond, to meet people on the borders, to demonstrate solidarity by offering what we could with the tools that we had as art therapists. For us, the work was a form of protest and action against the hostilities we saw aimed at refugees and migrants. By being present, we hoped to actively communicate a different narrative to that being portrayed by the UK's government and media. In addition to this motivation, the insufficient investment in the UK in mental health and wellbeing provisions, particularly for those who had been displaced and were seeking support, meant that job opportunities as art therapists in this area were scarce and highly competitive. When employment as an art therapist arose outside of the UK, it opened up the opportunity to work within a context that we both had some experience in and were passionate about.

CONTEXT

When the project began in 2016, Greece, as a consequence of the EU's 'Dublin Regulation', was carrying an unprecedented responsibility for the refugee population that were heading towards Europe from parts of Africa and the Middle East. By the time we left the project in June 2018, it was estimated that Greece was hosting over 60,000 refugees, many of whom were placed in ill-equipped and over-crowded mainland and island camps (UNHCR, 2020b).

In October 2016, the charity Flourish Foundation responded to this situation by visiting various refugee camps in Greece to explore if an art therapy service might be useful and one camp took this up. It was agreed that a large building at the back of the camp could be used for this purpose and a volunteer-based 8-week pilot project commenced. At the end of what seemed like a successful 8 weeks, Flourish Foundation secured funding from grants, private donors and fundraising events and was able to purchase a large Isobox to be used as an art studio, and to send a team of two UK-based art therapists to continue groups for men, women and children for a further 18 months.

The refugee camp was in a remote industrialised area situated on a disused army base. Initially it was considered an unofficial camp (not legally approved by local or national Greek authorities); many of the residents had arrived in May 2016 and spent months living in tents and shelters they had constructed with tarpaulin and found building materials. In October 2016 donated Isoboxes that had bunk beds, sinks and an air conditioning system transitioned the residents into safer shelter. The rows of numbered Isoboxes created a sense of order and authority; Figure 10.1 illustrates this change. Whilst the residents welcomed the safety and protection from the elements that the Isoboxes provided, there was also a sense of trepidation, distrust and uncertainty towards the change, with a fear that their asylum situation might become a permanent fixture.

In the camp, an intergovernmental organisation (IGO) held the responsibility of site management, shelter and coordination. During the day, the residents had access to medical assistance, hygiene utilities, clothing and food distributions, education, and some psychosocial services for women and children. Greek safeguarding officers and psychologists, employed by an IGO and non-governmental organisation (NGO), were also present on site. Flourish Foundation hosted regular

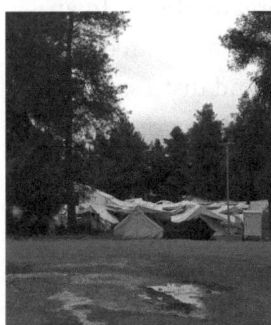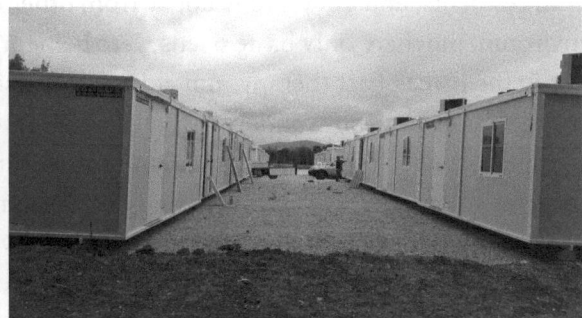

Figure 10.1 *Transition from tents to Isoboxes.*

meetings with the safeguarding officer and psychologist in order to discuss any concerns. Linking in with these professionals and other valuable on-site organisations also enabled us to signpost and share information with group members when needed.

From 2016 to 2018 the majority of people living in the camp were Syrian and Kurdish, with a smaller number of individuals from Africa and further areas of the Middle East. Numbers fluctuated between 600 and 900 residents, with roughly equal numbers across men, women and children.

THE ART STUDIO

The men's group was set up in the art studio with a central and communal table that was arranged with art materials, books and art postcards, and a separate area for refreshments. The largest wall was reserved for people to display their artworks. This created conversations around what was exhibited and what was not displayed. Those artworks not on the walls were stored in folders and boxes in a locked cabinet.

Initially, art materials were brought over from the UK by the charity and thereafter sourced from the local town. The studio was always well stocked and we found the art resources brought a mixture of responses from both other organisations in the camp and the residents. Although largely well received, the studio, art materials and our presence there felt to us, at times, to be met with confusion, anger and frustration from residents, and envy and jealousy from other organisations. In an environment where only basic needs were being met it felt difficult to justify the place of art therapy, and at times of crisis and distress we felt like useless artists and wondered what it was we were doing there. As art therapist Savneet Talwar describes, 'concepts of "art as healing" can only go so far when poverty is rampant and people do not have enough food to eat, clothes to wear or predictable shelter' (Talwar, 2019, pp. 6–7). The concept of art therapy was not easily translated to residents, or widely understood, and so finding the words to describe our service whilst also feeling uncertain of its value felt challenging.

Over the 18 months the art studio was broken into on a number of occasions. It seemed poignant that items were rarely taken. We felt that this was a communication about destitution and a desperate search for something more. The act of breaking-in left us feeling frustrated and unwanted, feelings perhaps familiar to many of the camp's residents.

At times the children would attack the exterior of the Isobox, acting out aggression and rage. They threw stones at the walls, windows and at us, rushing into the studio and attempting to hide under the tables. We tried to understand their anger and frustration as feelings evoked by yet another border. We considered that we might have been seen as hostile strangers enforcing rules and intruding into their home, a situation that many had experienced before.

It was therefore decided that the art studio would be locked, with the keys left in the door for people to leave. This meant that group members had to knock to gain entry and we would see people to the door to secure it once they had left. Whilst this helped to protect the space from being disturbed, it evoked in us uncomfortable feelings about our power and authority.

THE MEN'S ART THERAPY GROUP

Within the camp there were designated, safe and supported closed off spaces for women and children. These spaces provided opportunities for female residents to relax, socialise and receive information. The men, though, without designated places within services or projects available to them, tended to sit in small groups in exposed areas of the site. Before each session we walked through the refugee camp inviting residents to the art studio.

The men's art therapy sessions ran three times a week for two hours, at times with over 20 members accessing the space. The group was diverse, with men from different countries and ages spanning from 18 to over 70 years old. Group members would come and go in the men's groups, dropping in for a few minutes or staying for the two-hour duration. We wanted to create a space that was accessible and so flexibility was central to our approach. We would try to adapt to changes in the camp, such as sleeping patterns and cultural holidays, by adjusting the timetable to make the group more accessible.

Where we were conscious of them, we attempted to acknowledge cultural differences and attune with the community to avoid making Eurocentric assumptions (Kristel, 2013). Noting the physical and emotional strength that was demonstrated as the community pulled together against the inadequacies of the environment, we worked to welcome and generate a creative community in the art studio, one where an individual might find respite from the outside environment, and comfort and support from other members.

At times we noticed that the men made negative comments about other services, countries and political groups whilst positive comments were associated with the charity, the art studio and us. We wondered if splitting off anger associated with our limitations and failings functioned as a way to protect the space and continue a narrative of a good place. Perhaps the splitting served as a useful mechanism for making an unacceptable situation feel more acceptable.

For some of the group members the use of art materials was something new and required encouragement or advice. Prevailing depictions were of homes, landscapes and images made for, and of, loved ones. Many of the artworks created connections between group members as identities and experiences were shared with one another and expressed verbally within the group.

There is a lack of governmental responsibility towards refugees and asylum seekers across the globe; the UK, with its hostile environment policy, was, and is at the time of our writing, deliberately stalling asylum applications. In the group we would often hear descriptions and observe artwork that expressed feelings of being stuck and in limbo. In the men's group one member used clay to depict two figures falling and suspended in the air (Figure 10.2). We noted how the figures looked as though they were tumbling, reaching towards each other yet not quite touching. The fragile nature of the object meant that it broke and required the artist to glue the pieces back together. Looking at the physicality of the piece, it seems to mirror what we witnessed of the residents' experiences within the asylum system. The missing element of a depicted location in the artwork seems to reflect a sense of boundlessness, that these figures could be anywhere and nowhere. We are left wondering how and where they will land.

Without the use of interpreters, or a common language, we acknowledged our limitations in regard to understanding and exploring the group members' experiences verbally. The group was instead led by the most common language spoken in the room, at times this was English, Arabic, Kurmanji or the artwork. When conversations took place in a language different from ours we might ask if anyone could translate. At times this was not possible or we were told it did not matter. Sometimes a silence would ensue and we could be left with feelings of being shut out or misunderstood, and we wondered how these instances were experienced and understood by group members. Perhaps the silences articulated the unspeakable or were an opportunity for quiet reflection. The art, however,

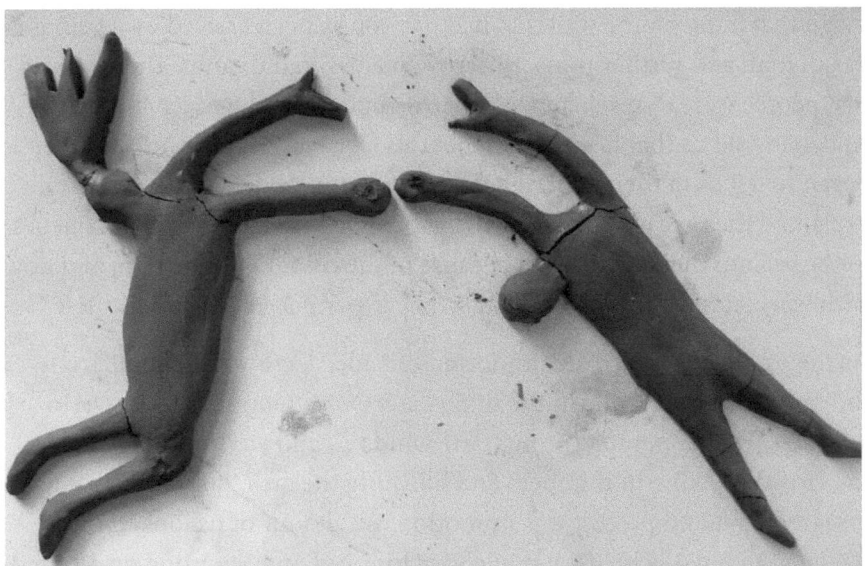

Figure 10.2 'Falling and suspended in air'. A group member's artwork.

continued to be created and was always a returning point of connection and a source of understanding.

VIGNETTES

The following vignettes are reflections on experiences that we feel demonstrate the asylum system as a hostile environment that induces complex and distressing experiences for those seeking safety. Through these accounts, we hope to illustrate the challenges we faced in holding and protecting a space that felt under threat, often drawing us and group members to the physical and psychological edge.

VIGNETTE 1

One afternoon two men from South Sudan joined the men's art group. To protect their anonymity we will refer to them as Abdallah and Zachariah. The camp had a small black African population at this time and we were aware of racist instances that had occurred within the camp towards some of the black residents. As we approached the end of the session, ourselves, Abdallah and Zachariah were left in the room. Zachariah commented on a sign that hung on the wall that had previously been created by a young Yazidi man and further transcribed by an elder in the camp. The sign said that people were to respect each other within the studio. Zachariah and Abdallah told us that it was good that this sign was in the room and they began to tell us of their experiences in the camp. Abdallah and Zachariah explained the racism they were facing, being pushed to the back of queues for buses into the nearby town because of the colour of their skin, and how each week, despite their complaints, they experienced the same issues.

As they spoke we heard a commotion outside. A crowd of people from the camp were gathering at the main gate. Our attention was drawn to see what was happening through the windows and we commented on the crowd growing in numbers and blocking the area. It seemed that a disagreement and protest was in motion. As all four of us looked on, a young man outside held a baton above his head and, standing on a raised path, shouted towards the crowd in an apparent gesture of incitement. Abdallah and Zachariah explained that, for them, seeing this type of event was a usual occurrence in the camp. As the crowd continued to gather nearer to the art studio, we, the therapists, made the decision that the session would need to end early. Our main exit was now blocked, leaving us feeling unsafe. We left the art studio all together and were met by a colleague from another organisation who told us that a protest was underway due to a disagreement between two families within the camp. They explained that the inciting gesture had apparently been a call for a divide between the Middle Eastern Arabs and the Kurds within the camp. We decided that for our safety we would leave the site for the day through another exit. After explaining this to Abdallah and Zachariah, we watched them walk away through the Isoboxes and then we left.

Reflection

In prioritising our own safety we experienced feelings of shame and guilt. We left the camp that day questioning our role and feeling powerless and useless in such difficult circumstances. We acknowledged that our position meant we could decide when to end the session, seemingly controlling the border in and out of the art studio and reinstating a separateness and authority between us and the group members.

Reflecting on our responses, we considered the behaviour and events that we had witnessed. We wondered if the young Kurdish man with the baton was re-enacting his past experiences of violence, segregation and prejudice – perhaps the environment pushed him to his psychological edge and he had become unable to contain his feelings any longer. We wondered how it felt for the young man to command power at this point and to call for division within the community, and, when the protest ended, how it felt for him to then return to this community.

We also considered what it might be like for Abdallah and Zachariah to be seeking safety from violent prejudice only to continue to witness and experience it in a place of so-called refuge. We wondered how they felt that day as we closed the art studio. Had it been enough for them to voice their feelings about what they were facing? Had the closure of the studio that day and the prioritising of our safety been another experience for them of being pushed to the back of the queue or of unresolved complaint, and in this, were we, too, a part of the inadequate system?

We considered our whiteness, nationality and femaleness and what it might represent to them, particularly in light of the UK's history of colonialism in South Sudan that has tragically impacted its political situation. Our white privilege allowed us to move between borders around the world with little interjection or experience of imposing limits, despite our nation's violent and oppressive history. We felt shame and guilt at our privilege and our freedom to leave the camp to find safety elsewhere.

In our next meeting with camp management we raised the experiences of racism that Abdallah and Zachariah had brought to the session. These conversations about racism in the camp were ongoing at the time we left.

VIGNETTE 2

Once a week the Isobox next to the art studio was occupied by an IGO offering legal advice. Arriving in the camp on this day we witnessed residents outside this Isobox holding a piece of paper with a number scribbled on it that marked their place in the queue. Each week we were reminded of the waiting game that is the immobilising and intrinsic experience of being displaced in a refugee camp. As Pai (2018) expresses, 'Refugees and migrants caught up in the managed migration system of the EU are seen and dealt with as simply figures on the balance sheets of the asylum reception chain – their needs and aspirations often treated as irrelevant' (Pai, 2018, p. 13).

On this particular day the art therapy studio felt like a waiting room. Whilst some group members came to the doorway to inform us of their place in the queue, others, knowing they had a long wait, came in to use the art materials and sit with other group members, perhaps partially alleviating the anxiety and boredom of waiting.

The repercussions associated with the legal advice meetings would often be brought into the art studio. Feelings of having a constant place in a queue, being pushed to the back whilst others seemingly jumped in front, and the disbelief at receiving asylum appointment dates scheduled for over a year's time were just some of the issues expressed within the sessions.

On this day we began to hear a commotion outside the Isobox. The group's attention was drawn away from the art making and one group member got up to see what was happening. On opening the door, we were met with a man in distress holding a bag. The group members stepped outside the space to talk to him as we stood in the doorway watching and witnessing the interaction. Unsure whether to keep hold of the now empty space inside or become part of the interaction outside, we remained on the threshold.

The man spoke of how his home had been bombed, leaving him with multiple injuries. He repeated the phrase, 'words, words, words, no action', in English and began to shake the bag upside down, emptying the contents onto the gravel in front of us. Paper documents, packets of medication and multiple hospital x-rays fell to the ground.

Some of the group members and the art therapist closest to the man stepped down from the doorway to help him pick up his belongings, whilst the other therapist stayed in the doorway. As his items were gathered up, we could see what the content of the bag was exposing. It held testimony to the realities of war; evidence of bombs that devastate and the wounds that are inflicted. Handing his belongings back to him, the man thanked the group and walked away from the Isobox. The rest of the group then thanked us for the session and left.

Reflection

When we returned inside the Isobox we sat with the artwork left on the table. What initially struck us was how the work appeared as if abandoned and without conclusion. In the moment, our attempts to make meaning of this incident felt inhibited by feelings of grief and rage at the situation.

On reflection, we began to think about this experience in relation to re-enactment.

Herman writes that often people who have experienced trauma relive the moment (of the trauma) in thoughts, dreams and their actions. She goes on to say that 'adults as well as children often feel impelled to re-create the moment of terror, either in literal or disguised form' (Herman, 2015, p. 39). She describes these re-enactments as having a feeling of involuntariness and that they can be thought about as spontaneous attempts to integrate the traumatic event. The man's act of throwing down his personal belongings felt like a bomb being dropped. In exposing his medical records and personal belongings in this way, he seemed to demonstrate the abuse and humiliation he was experiencing in needing to prove he was deserving of asylum after surviving a bombing attack.

The abrupt ending of the session and abandoned artwork spoke to us about the lives the group members had been abruptly forced to abandon but also how they may feel abandoned by the international community, stuck in the camp and waiting. The act of putting away the artwork after the incident allowed us to contain the feelings we were left with of a session that had ended abruptly and unexpectedly; it also seemed to mirror the picking up and putting away of the man's belongings outside.

It seemed that the group members could not bear to stay inside and ignore what was happening outside. As therapists we questioned whether we should have stayed inside, holding the space, however like the men, we also could not bear to be bystanders.

Witnessing the situation from our position in the camp, we saw the powerful influence that the residents had on one another, both inside and outside of the art studio. The man outside was able to share his distress and the group members responded to him. Perhaps this helped to provide a sense of connectivity and restore a sense of a meaningful world (Herman, 2015). We hoped that seeing the community respond to him with empathy and compassion carried an active message of support and hope for the future.

DISCUSSION

The reinforcement of global borders has charged a racist rhetoric towards migration, perpetuating the dehumanising and divisive idea of who is in and who is out. During our time working in the camp, we witnessed that whilst their asylum applications are processed, people seeking asylum are often left on a threshold and dependent on a dysfunctional system.

Writing this chapter has been an exploration and opportunity to revisit our time in the refugee camp and to explore and challenge our perceptions, approaches and intentions. We have looked at the influence of aspects of our identities on the work and considered the impacts of these on an environment where people are politicised.

Part of this writing process led us to look back at the artwork we made in the men's groups alongside the group members. Our own art making informed our work within the groups and increased our understanding of our feelings and responses to the environment and situation we were witnessing. As Allen (2007, p. 75) notes, the art therapist's images can inform us of the dysfunctions of the system we work in and deepen our understanding of the clients' experiences.

When we returned to the UK we observed our images together and were struck by the amount of circular artworks we had created within the men's groups (Figure 10.3). During our discussions Katie observed the circles as a narrative, one that was cyclical, like a vicious circle out of which there often seemed no end. At times, as illustrated in Figure 10.3, shards or lines surrounded or penetrated the circles, which Emily felt expressed a collective feeling of intrusion. We reflected on this as representing part of what we had heard of the experiences of the residents' lives being intruded upon and becoming fragmented, and also in relation to our experiences of the studio being broken into. We both commented on the circle as representing the inside and outside of the refugee camp environment, and the line it drew seemed to be the 'edge' that the residents and the art studio occupied.

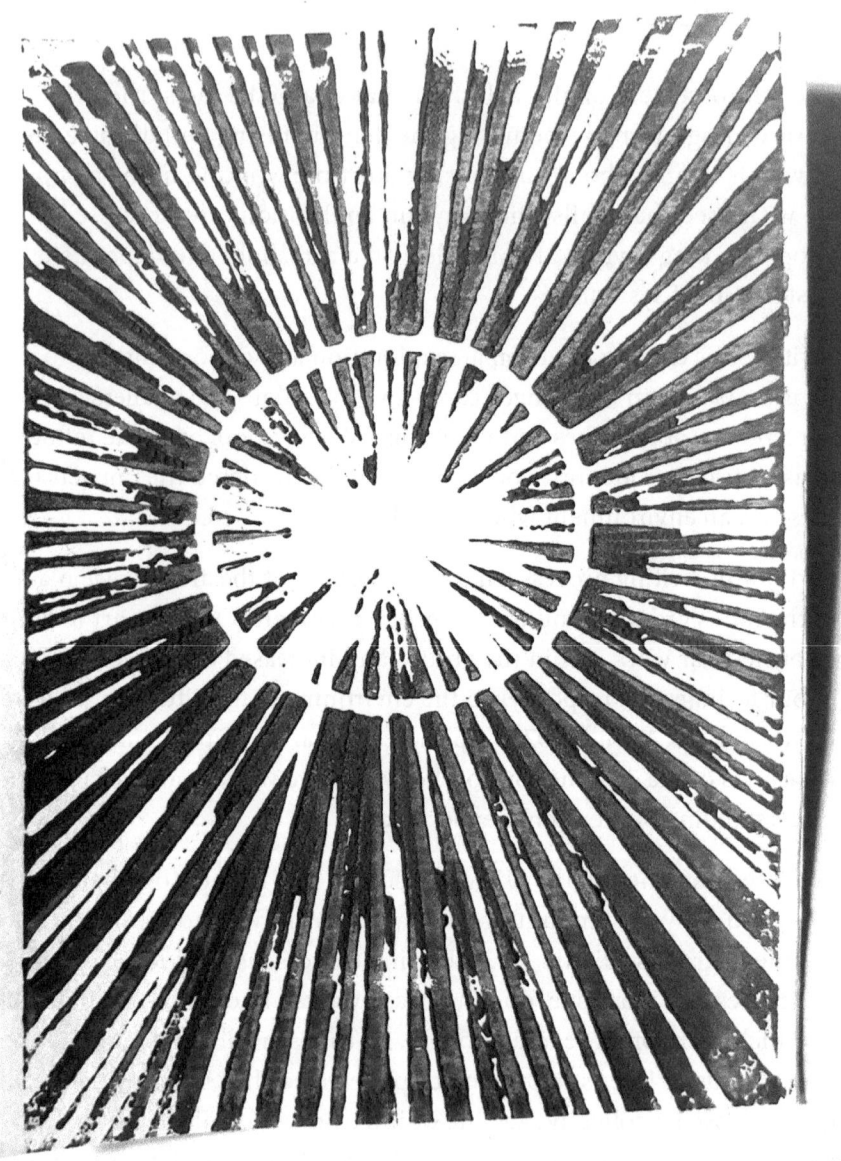

Figure 10.3 '*Circles*'. *An art therapist's artwork.*

Through the vignettes we aimed to portray what we felt were some of the impacts of the refugee camp and the asylum system on people's lives and wellbeing. What we witnessed within these two encounters were situations where people were pushed to their limits by the asylum system and the hostile environment it creates.

Working in this environment, at times, left us feeling useless, stuck and ambivalent about our position in the camp. Whilst we could see the value of the art studio and its ability to counter some of the negative effects of this inhospitable environment, we also questioned if we could be contributing to a form of 'inoculation' against an 'ill system' (Allen, 2007) that encouraged the residents to be more accepting of the unacceptable conditions.

It seemed to us, however, that the act of art making poignantly countered the oppressive and dehumanising environment, and fulfilled the need that group members sought out to regain autonomy and restore a sense of purpose and humanity. The very action of *doing* was in opposition to the system, which stalled, and the feelings of being stuck that the group members expressed. The art studio was an inclusive space which facilitated an experience of belonging, restored purpose, and allowed for the collective witnessing of experiences inside, outside and on the edge of the room. This, with the commonality within the artworks, fostered a sense of solidarity.

In writing this chapter we have come to realise the significance of witnessing the edge. Whether it is where people are placed geographically or pushed to in their tolerance, the edges are a place of uncertainty and where much of our work took place.

As we approached the end of this chapter it also became apparent that, for us, there was a dichotomy within our work. Whilst the service had high levels of engagement, we were often left questioning the purpose of art therapy and our presence there. Yet it was within these lines of uncertainty that we felt the work took place and, in the end, it was in tolerating both the impossible *and* possible that the work within this hostile system was able to thrive.

REFERENCES

Allen, P.B. (2007). Wielding the Shield. In: Kaplan, F. (ed.), *Art Therapy and Social Action*. 1st ed., London and New York: Jessica Kingsley Publishers, pp. 72–85.

Herman, J.L. (2015). *Trauma and Recovery: The Aftermath of Violence: From Domestic Abuse to Political Terror*. 1st ed., New York: Basic Books, pp. 33–73.

Kristel, J. (2013). The Process of Attunement between Therapist and Client. In: Howie, P., Prasad, S. and Kristel, J. (eds), *Using Art Therapy with Diverse Populations*. 1st ed., London: Jessica Kingsley Publishers, pp. 85–94.

Pai, H. (2018). *Bordered Lives: How Europe Fails Refugees and Migrants*. 1st ed., Oxford: New Internationalist Publications, p. 13.

Talwar, S.K. (2019). Beyond Multiculturalism and Cultural Competence. In: *Art Therapy For Social Justice: Radical Intersections*. 1st ed., New York: Routledge, pp. 6–7.

Trilling, D. (2018). *Lights in the Distance: Exile and Refuge at the Borders of Europe*. 1st ed., London: Picador, p. 241.

UNHCR (2020a). *Asylum in the UK*. Available at: https://www.unhcr.org/uk/asylum-in-the-uk.html [Accessed 15th January 2019].

UNHCR (2020b). *Greece*. Available at: https://www.unhcr.org/uk/greece.html [Accessed 4th June 2020].

Politics in action

Sally Skaife and Jon Martyn

DOI: 10.4324/9781003107408-14

'The law locks up the man or woman
Who steals the goose from off the common
But leaves the greater villain loose
Who steals the common from the goose'

Eighteenth-century protest poem against the enclosures
of the common land. Author unknown.

THE WORLD IS ON FIRE

It is becoming increasingly urgent that there is effective opposition to neoliberalism since the pursuit of profit threatens us with climate extinction. Discontent has led to neo-fascist 'populist' leaders taking power, exploiting social division and further denigrating the working class, attacking our already flawed democracies and threatening war. We now know that our increasing plunder of the world's resources is putting us in danger of further crises, with more pandemics and ecological collapse, yet onward we go. How should art therapy groups be run in a time of mass resistance, as this should surely become?

For art therapy to be a practice in which individual suffering is understood as inextricably related to a political system that causes suffering whilst it makes individual victims feel responsible for their own plight, there has to be resistance to that system built into the practice. The question is, how can this be possible when, as we have seen in the chapters in this book, if we can keep our art therapy spaces at all, it is nigh impossible to keep them free from intrusion by antithetical neoliberal agendas and ideologies. We have suggested that any progress relies on the exposure of the contradictions thrown up by neoliberalism. Contradictions in art therapy might include the following: creating a need through constructing patients as having a lack, and then creating a product to meet that need – art as empowerment; with manualised approaches like mentalisation based therapy (MBT), we purport to know the outcome before we begin, which presents a contradiction with the idea that through art making, art therapy gives agency to the client; lastly, how can the art therapist meet the requirements of the institution where those appear in contradiction to the needs of the people the group serves? We are suggesting that we engage with the neoliberal intrusions rather than attempt to ignore them. If the contradictions are made overt, there's the possibility that the group engages in something akin to political action in their attempts to make sense of them. In this chapter we explore the way contradictions emerged in some of the chapters. We develop the idea of the art therapy group as a heterotopic space, which opens up a possibility for play with different experiences, in which we can be positioned differently whilst recognising current realities. Empowerment, then, is through a process of collective creation of the space, an art therapy group practice that is a political praxis.

As we have seen in the preceding chapters, there are many threats to the art therapy space. Firstly, privatisation has led to a massive loss of publicly owned space. Starved of funds from the government, councils are forced to sell off their remaining communal spaces to raise money for essential services in the borough. In inner cities there is a process of gentrification, with poor people being pushed out to the periphery. The neglect of housing, such as Grenfell Tower in North Kensington and Chelsea, has been a deliberate policy to enable the buying up of the land for the lucrative sale of private property. In Chapter Nine, the building in which the art therapy studio was held was being sold, and the women's prison in Chapter Eight was put up for sale and the prisoners displaced. Chapter Four, though, describes resistance to this trend in the takeover of a Community Centre by the community to which it belonged only in name.

Secondly, art therapy groups are threatened by the precarity of the art therapist's employment. Gone are the permanent full-time contracts of the past – art therapists are most often employed sessionally, on short-term contracts, or work privately. This means that they have no job security, will often be in debt and live with wage insecurity. It is no surprise that 90% of the profession are women. The art therapist's insecure position makes a long-term art therapy group process difficult to maintain. Whereas there was often a gulf between the paid therapist and the paying (even if through taxation) client, now art therapists might well be as poor and insecure as their clients (Watts et al., 2018). With this, empathy might well be replaced by solidarity, suggesting a different sort of therapeutic relationship.

Third, the art therapy group is intruded on by neoliberal agendas antithetical to it, not only in the form of measurement and audit, as described in Chapter Two, but also in the way staff groups are set up to be in competition. For example, in Chapter Eight, the art therapist felt unsupported by prison officers, and in Chapter Six, the difficulties that arose between the teachers and the art therapists had a competitive edge.

Fourth, increased inequality (Wilkinson and Pickett, 2010) in income and wealth, and increased struggle around issues of race and gender, citizenship rights and of housing and work insecurity, lead inevitably to increased potential for conflicts within art therapy groups. This was apparent in Chapter Seven on the acute ward. The doctor's surprise at the fragility of the group when, in response to his and his entourage's appearance, members hurriedly left, exposed a gulf between his personal experience and that of group members. At the time of writing, we face further incursions in keeping with so-called populism; the government is proposing a series of acts which grant police impunity, criminalise public protest, criminalise our Gypsy/Romany/Traveller communities and further negate migrant rights.

Lastly, much of NHS mental health care is now being carried out in the private sector, and current government plans, under the misleading banner of 'Integrated Care Systems', will increasingly place the whole of the NHS under the control of transnational corporations whose shareholders can make profit from them, copying US Health Maintenance Organisations. Thus, privatisation means that many art therapy groups' primary purpose will be to create profit for shareholders; this puts them at odds with the requirements of their members, creating contradictions that are irreconcilable without political change, as we have discussed. Similarly, many schools have been acadamised and are now owned by, and run as, businesses, with pupils, parents, teachers and the local community having very little control. When the art therapists in Chapter

Six met with teachers, the difficulty the management had with accepting that the children might be affected by the fire seemed related to its inconvenience to the school's purpose.

In response to these threats, art therapy groups have sometimes been created outside of traditional institutions, where it has been easier to create appropriate spaces and to work on one's own terms. Where the practitioners have a political perspective, this has often involved interventions at community level. However, because it is impossible to separate any art therapy group from the systems in which they take place, this cannot in itself be enough. There is also the factor, described by Blackwell (2003) and Layton (2019), of white therapists having ingrained in them, at an unconscious level, a sense that they deserve their privilege gained through skin colour and thus are likely to ignore injustice meted out against black people. If this were not so, it would not have taken the filmed death of George Floyd in 2020 for large numbers of white people to join the Black Lives Matter demonstrations. A key factor in the continuation of police brutality towards black people is that the white population has ignored it. With all these factors, how are we to build resistance to the system into our art therapy group practice?

We have suggested in previous chapters that we need to take hold of the contradictions that capitalism gives rise to. In Chapter Three, we suggested that dialectics and deconstruction might be tools that could be applied in art therapy to work with the inevitable contradictions and binaries that emerge in our practice. We thought that mind/body divisions exploited for political reasons in gender, race and class, were also there in art therapy practice in the division between talking, or the therapeutic relationship, and making art in therapy, all being binaries that can be deconstructed.

We see in the chapters involving art therapy practice how contradictions are powerfully held in the artwork. The wounded bear that is on the front cover of the book, without its words, 'Don't fuck with the wounded bear' (the expletive was thought to present an impediment to sales if it were on the front cover), is both a victim and a dangerous threat. The bear deconstructs the binary of perpetrator/victim by showing us that the wounded animal will become enraged when they are 'cut'. As the artist Andrew Mead makes clear, this refers to austerity and cuts to public services.

The child's rainbow drawing in Chapter Six, shaped like a tower, frames the absence of the community's distress, commenting on the school's request that the fire at the tower was not mentioned so that everything could be kept nice, like a rainbow (without the rain). In Chapter Ten, the asylum seeker empties his bag onto the ground, revealing personal, bodily related items, in an act that demonstrates his bodily subjugation. In order to gain asylum he must turn his torture into the right sort of data, payment for the hope that the violence will end. With the Grenfell anniversary banner in Chapter Five, a question is raised as to whether it is a protest banner to be permanently displayed or a product of art therapy.

The contradictions will be there whether we look at them or not, but art psychodynamic group spaces allow for this exposure; attempts made at reconciling them involve the participants in a political process. We can see this happening in Chapter Nine in the contradiction of a community space that was run by therapists, which posed questions as to who should protect the space when the service was threatened. The deconstruction of the inevitable binaries – of race, gender and other systems of domination – can expose what gets hidden by dominant voices. One side of the binary only exists because of the other, as summed up in the question asked by James Baldwin, 'why do white people need the negro?'

We thought these deconstructions might be ways in which art therapy could be envisioned as a political practice and that, therefore, it was a good lens to think about art therapy literature written by those art therapists who were interested in creating the same. We found that some of them were thinking differently, and this might have been because our discourse is necessarily particular to our context, or because the work mainly involved interventions at a community level and/or short-term work. We noted contradictions, mainly that the role of the therapist was not discussed in the papers we looked at. In some papers, where the projects entailed leaving the art therapy space to go on demonstrations or to exhibit work, roles were deconstructed through this action: there were puppeteers, political protesters and exhibiting artists in place of clients. This disruption invites us to think in new ways about art therapy spaces.

WHAT IS MEANT BY HETEROTOPIC SPACES?

Chapter Three described the Art Therapy Large Group on the MA Art Psychotherapy programme at Goldsmiths, University of London, as a Foucauldian heterotopic space (Skaife et al., 2020). It is a space which feels as if it exists outside of time, that brings together in a single real place other spaces, that in themselves are incompatible. Foucault gives the theatre as a paradigmatic example. Issues belonging to these other spaces are reproduced, re-enacted and performed, thus deepening meaning and understanding. In this 'play space', glimpses are had of alternative ways of doing living, though the space is also disturbing.

The French philosopher Henri Lefebvre described heterotopic space rather differently. Where Foucault's spaces are enclosed, for example, ships, boarding schools and the traditional theatre space, Lefebvre envisages liminal social spaces of possibility in ordinary, everyday life, in which 'something different', a disruption to the usual order, can emerge. 'This "something different" does not necessarily arise out of a conscious plan, but more simply out of what people do, feel, sense, and come to articulate as they seek meaning in their daily lives' (Harvey, 2012, p. xvii). Lefebvre sees the revolutionary moment as 'the spontaneous coming together in a moment of "irruption;" when disparate heterotopic groups suddenly see, if only for a fleeting moment, the possibilities of collective action to create something radically different' (ibid). Lefebvre's ideas suggest that group acts of dissent, such as demonstrations, pickets or occupations, in their disruption of neoliberal relations, are potent heterotopic spaces. They offer opportunity to transcend politically constructed divisions in race, gender, age, disability and class, aiding the recognition of differences in positionality, thus enabling fleeting experiences of empowerment and solidarity.

Heterotopic spaces will be objects of repression by the state in the interests of capital, but such repression also generates possible further heterotopias. In the art therapy group, there is a dynamic of destabilisation of art therapy group boundaries, as we saw in Chapter Nine, and the challenge art therapists face is to develop an agility of boundary keeping which needs both plasticity and reinforcement. An example of this is the fate of material artworks produced in therapy.

Art has always been able to be taken out of the space and recontextualised. The pioneering art therapist Edward Adamson took artworks made by patients to the psychiatrist to aid in the construction of the patients' diagnosis, but he also exhibited the artwork with the intention of destigmatising that diagnosis. In the literature reviewed in Chapter Three, Tillet and Tillet (2018) describe artwork being taken to a protest, and 'Najma' et al. (2021) discuss asylum seekers exploring their artistic identity through exhibiting and selling work. In Chapter Six, artwork from the classroom was taken to the management to demonstrate that the art therapy group was providing a space for the working through of distress. In Chapter Nine, studio members display their artwork to convey their discontent to management. It has been the tradition though, in most UK art therapy, that the art therapist keeps the work securely in the studio in order to protect the separate 'as if' space of the therapy. This flexibility with boundaries, now becoming more mainstream as many art therapy groups go online, with the result that artwork is kept in the client's home rather than by the therapist, seems to be a response to the 'threats' described above. A question is raised as to whether this change adds to the erosion of the therapeutic space or whether it creates different political possibilities. Are these mutually exclusive ideas? Does the fantasy collapse when action is taken? Is the maintenance of fantasy a disavowal of material reality? With appropriate boundaries, these contradictions can be ones which the group grapples with. The removal of art from the therapy space to educate those outside it has parallels with the revolutionary work of the Martinique psychiatrist Frantz Fanon.

Fanon, who was one of the first to write about the mental health effects of imperialism and racism, devoted himself to community psychiatry and then to the anti-colonial struggle in Algeria. He said that a patient has to first treat the organisation in which they are in before that organisation can treat them (Fanon, 2018).

Can we foresee a situation in which the art therapy group starts out by questioning, challenging and treating its institutional base? Fanon's notion of the institution needing to be treated *before* it can treat the patient suggests that this boundary between the inside and the outside of the therapy space is made present right at the beginning. If illusion and disavowal, and projection of its pathology onto the individual, is the sickness of neoliberalism, the therapist has to facilitate a process of liberation that threatens the institutional ground on which the therapist and the group stand. This will potentially enable the clients to rid themselves of the stigma and sickness that has been projected onto them.

Fanon's emphasis on the psychoanalytic notion of introjection is important here. It is a recognition of how the outside world impinges on the internal world at an unconscious level. This has been termed in group analysis as the 'social unconscious' (Hopper, 2003), a term which has been interpreted in various different ways since Hopper introduced it in 2003 (Hopper and Weinberg, 2011, 2018). However, the concept of intersubjectivity, developed by Heidegger, Merleau-Ponty and other Continental philosophers, understands any separation of inner and outer worlds as based on an essentialist idea of identity. The implication of intersubjectivity is that all therapy, from the start, has as its subject an individually embodied political world, and thus it cannot help but have an impact on that world. The artwork is a transitional object in this sense. It is both a visual response to a cultural world and, as a tangible piece, has within it the possibility, even if never realised, of having an impact on the cultural world beyond the group. Indeed, it has an impact on the artist themselves and the other group members, and through this, the world. Here the separation of the personal and political, which is the bedrock of neoliberal ideology, is eroded.

Heterotopic spaces, which do not attempt to tidy up contradictions and allow the inevitable conflicts brought into the group via the threats to have presence, allow for new possibilities to be worked out collectively. As they disrupt the established order of things they will be unsettling, confusing and disturbing. As shown in Dudley's group in Chapter Three and Lambert's group in Chapter Five, conflicts open the opportunity to form a collective body of resistance. The intrusion by the doctor and team on the acute ward group in Chapter Seven was a threat that one of the patients upturned when he told the art therapist that if she allied with the psychiatrist, he would never return to the group. This disturbance to the normal order gave the client a fleeting moment in which he became an employer threatening to 'sack' the art therapist.

The Kapitan et al. (2011), Tillet and Tillet (2018) and 'Najma' et al. (2021) papers suggest that the art therapy groups are kept as 'safe spaces', with the disruption happening only outside of them back in home communities, on the demonstration, or at the exhibition. Chapter Eight describes the disruption in a prison art therapy group that is so disturbing that the group has to be closed. Here it seems that the institution's desire to punish, enacting society's bullying contempt for working-class women, is powerfully projected into the group. Where care and punishment are overtly confused, this heterotopia seems impossible to manage. For a therapeutic heterotopia to emerge, the boundaries must have the sort of flexibility that allows both for the presence of conflict to be reworked creatively and to be recognised as belonging in the political dynamics to which we are all subject, and the maintenance of a space which ensures that no real harm is done. Violence is present, or latent, in all political struggle, but it has no place in a therapy group.

Thinking of art therapy spaces as heterotopic gives us an answer to Waller's question as to whether or not we are still pragmatic rebels (Waller, 2004), a question she asked at the 2018 BAAT AGM after relating points from her inaugural lecture. We say that pragmatism is necessarily a collusion with the establishment, and one that should only be used with working class emancipation in mind. The video of George Floyd's murder in Minneapolis can help us think about this.

In going viral the video transported a violent murder around the world so that its horror and injustice could be felt by all who saw it. The resultant global outrage, expressed in Black Lives Matter demonstrations, has led the London-based *International Journal of Art Therapy* (*IJAT*) to recognise the exclusionary nature of its editorial rules and to make valuable reforms. These changes are encouraging, and we must remember that change came about through members who articulated discontent and laboured to develop decolonised standards. Similar attempts at decolonisation are happening in many organisations. Here positive change has come about quite quickly as a result of a disruption, with echoes of Lefebvre's discussion of disruptions in heterotypic spaces, and is ricocheting. This stands in contrast to the sort of pragmatism, as described in Chapter Two, that is driven by the market.

Back in 2001, Naomi Klein argued for a reclaiming of the commons, a need for thousands of local movements in which people fight for prosaic things, such as how often the bins are collected, stand up against police violence, against rent increases, for improving schools. All these, though, must be held under one massive global movement against the forced implementation of neoliberalism. She referred to the Zapatistas, an indigenous resistance group in Mexico, who named this 'one world with many worlds in it' (Hsiao and Lim, 2020, p. 322). She argues that we need to trust in people's ability to make the rules themselves and to make decisions that are best for them. Neoliberalism is biased at every level towards centralisation, waging a war on diversity. Many art therapy books end with ideas for what art therapists should do. We argue for the opposite and against models of art therapy. Instead, what is suggested by heterotopic spaces is that groups, with therapists responsive to contradictions and boundaries, should decide their own direction.

We are in need of heterotopic spaces to collectively imagine new possibilities and to work out how and where 'pragmatism' sits in relation to the urgent need to 'rebel', which will be a matter for tactics on the ground. We ask, who owns art therapy? A question which seeks to reveal the class interests that underlie our professional field. The question serves as a reminder that our practice is ultimately owned by us, its members. And without our clients, we would not need to exist. Therefore, we must ask each other, What do we stand for? Who do we stand with? And what do we oppose? To explore these questions can help us to develop the tools of resistance.

We are not arguing in this book for all our readers to become revolutionaries: the dynamics we have tried to describe, which promote the kind of agility in running groups that we are advocating, comes from the progress of neoliberal capitalism itself. All that is required is faith in the power of the art therapy process, faith in the group members, faith in the future, despite the present dire outlook for humanity, and an appropriate humility ...

REFERENCES

Blackwell, D. (2003). Colonialism and globalization: A group-analytic perspective. *Group Analysis*, 36(4), pp. 445–463.

Fanon, F. (2018). *Alienation and Freedom*. S. Corcoran (trans), J. Khalfa and R.J.C. Young (eds). London: Bloomsbury.

Harvey, D. (2012). *Rebel Cities: From the Right to the City to the Urban Revolution*. London and New York: Verso Books.

Hopper, E. (2003). *The Social Unconscious: Selected Papers* (Vol. 22). London and Philadelphia: Jessica Kingsley Publishers.

Hopper, E. and Weinberg, H. (eds) (2011). *The Social Unconscious in Persons, Groups and Societies, Volume 1: Mainly Theory*. London: Karnac Books.

Hopper, E. and Weinberg, H. (eds) (2018). *The Social Unconscious in Persons, Groups and Societies: Volume 1: Mainly Theory*. London and New York: Routledge.

Hsiao, A. and Lim, A. (2020). *The Verso Book of Dissent*. London and New York: Verso Books.

Kapitan, L., Litell, M. and Torres, A. (2011). Creative art therapy in a community's participatory research and social transformation. *Art Therapy*, 28(2), pp. 64–73.

Klein, N. (2001). *No Logo*. Canada: Knopf Picador. First published 1999.

Layton, L. (2019). Transgenerational hauntings: Toward a social psychoanalysis and an ethic of dis-illusionment. *Psychoanalytic Dialogues*, 29(2), pp. 105–121.

'Najma', Kaczynski, T., Martyn, J. and Hollamby, E. (2021). Image, Narrative and Migration. In: West, J. (ed.), *Using Image and Narrative in Therapy for Trauma, Addiction and Recovery*. London and Philadelphia: Jessica Kingsley Publishers, pp. 282–297.

Skaife, S., Morris, L., Tipple, R. and Velada, D. (2020). The story of the camera, a case study of an art therapy large group. *Group Analysis*, 53(1), pp. 37–59.

Tillet, S. and Tillet, S. (2018). 'You Want to Be Well?': Self-Care as a Black Feminist Intervention in Art Therapy. In: Talwar, S. (ed.), *Art Therapy for Social Justice*. London and New York: Routledge, pp. 123–143.

Waller, D. (2004). *Art Therapists: Pragmatic Rebels*. Goldsmiths College, University of London.

Watts, P., Gilfillan, P. and de Zárate, M.H. (2018). Art therapy and poverty: Examining practitioners' experiences of working with children and young people in areas of multiple deprivation in West Central Scotland. *International Journal of Art Therapy*, 23(4), pp. 146–155.

Wilkinson, R. and Pickett, K. (2010). *The Spirit Level: Why Equality is Better for Everyone*. London: Penguin.

INDEX

Note: *Italic* page numbers refer to figures and photographs and page numbers followed by "n" denote footnotes.

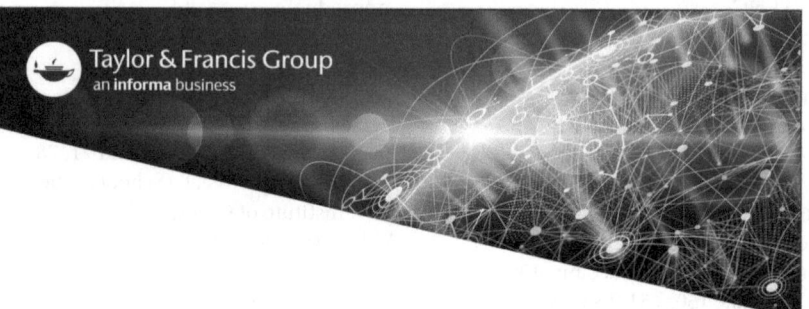
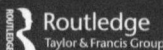
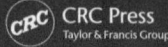